SAFE PASSAGE

A Guide for Addressing School Violence

SAFE PASSAGE
A Guide for Addressing School Violence

Edited by

Michael B. Kelly, M.D.
Anne B. McBride, M.D.

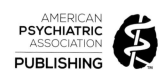

AMERICAN
PSYCHIATRIC
ASSOCIATION
PUBLISHING

If you wish to buy 50 or more copies of the same title, please go to www.appi.org/specialdiscounts for more information.

Copyright © 2020 American Psychiatric Association Publishing

ALL RIGHTS RESERVED

First Edition

Manufactured in the United States of America on acid-free paper
23 22 21 20 19   5 4 3 2 1

American Psychiatric Association Publishing
800 Maine Avenue SW
Suite 900
Washington, DC 20024-2812
www.appi.org

Library of Congress Cataloging-in-Publication Data
Names: Kelly, Michael B. (Professor of psychiatry), editor. | McBride, Anne B., editor. | American Psychiatric Association, issuing body.
Title: Safe passage : a guide for addressing school violence / edited by Michael B. Kelly and Anne B. McBride.
Other titles: Safe passage (Kelly)
Description: Second edition. | Washington, D.C. : American Psychiatric Association Publishing, [2020] | Includes bibliographical references.
Identifiers: LCCN 2019020784 (print) | ISBN 9781615370771 (paperback) ; (alk. paper) | ISBN 9781615372669 (ebook)
Subjects: MESH: Violence—prevention & control | Adolescent Behavior | Schools | Dangerous Behavior | Risk Assessment—methods | Bullying—prevention & control | United States
Classification: LCC RJ506.V56 (print) | LCC RJ506.V56 (ebook) | NLM WS 470.A4 | DDC 616.85/8200835—dc23

British Library Cataloguing in Publication Data
A CIP record is available from the British Library.

To Amelia, Conor, and baby brother: wishing you safe passage through rough seas and resilience in the face of adversity.

M.B.K.

To Maximus, Ernest, and Oscar: you inspire me to find safe passage for all.

A.B.M.

Contents

PART I
Foundations

Michael B. Kelly, M.D.
Anne B. McBride, M.D.
Arany Uthayakumar, B.A.
Jeff Bostic, M.D., Ed.D.
Sharon Hoover, Ph.D.

Michael B. Kelly, M.D.
Anne B. McBride, M.D.
Jeff Bostic, M.D., Ed.D.
Sharon Hoover, Ph.D.
Ana DiRago, Ph.D.
Arany Uthayakumar, B.A.

PART II
Threat and Risk Assessment

PART III
Interventions

Contributors

Amy Barnhorst, M.D.
Associate Professor of Clinical Psychiatry and Vice Chair of Community Psychiatry, Department of Psychiatry and Behavioral Sciences, University of California, Davis, Davis, California

Jeff Bostic, M.D., Ed.D.
Professor of Clinical Psychiatry, Department of Psychiatry, MedStar Georgetown University Hospital, Washington, DC

Tim Brennan, M.D., M.P.H.
Assistant Professor of Psychiatry; Director, Addiction Institute at Mt. Sinai West and St. Luke's Hospitals; Director, Fellowship in Addiction Medicine Program, Icahn School of Medicine at Mt. Sinai, New York, New York

Ana DiRago, Ph.D.
Clinical Instructor, Department of Psychiatry and Behavioral Sciences Stanford University School of Medicine, Stanford, California

Sharon Hoover, Ph.D.
Associate Professor, Division of Child and Adolescent Psychiatry, University of Maryland School of Medicine, Baltimore, Maryland

Michael B. Kelly, M.D.
Senior Psychiatrist, California Department of State Hospitals-Coalinga, Coalinga, California

Anne B. McBride, M.D.
Assistant Professor of Clinical Psychiatry and Program Director, Child and Adolescent Psychiatry Residency, Department of Psychiatry and Behavioral Sciences, University of California, Davis, Davis, California

Sophie Rosseel, M.D.
Psychiatry Resident, PGYII, Department of Psychiatry and Biobehavioral Sciences, University of California, Los Angeles, Los Angeles, California

Suzanne Shimoyama, M.D.
Assistant Professor of Clinical Psychiatry, Department of Psychiatry and Behavioral Sciences, University of California, Davis, Davis, California

Kelli Marie Smith, M.D.
Resident in Psychiatry, Department of Psychiatry and Behavioral Sciences, Stanford University School of Medicine, Stanford, California

Amy Toig, B.A.
Doctoral student in Clinical Psychology, Pacific Graduate School of Psychology, Palo Alto University, Stanford, California

Marcia Unger, M.D, M.P.H.
Child and Adolescent Psychiatry Resident, Department of Psychiatry and Behavioral Sciences, University of California, Davis, Davis, California

Arany Uthayakumar, B.A.
Editorial and Research Intern, Department of Psychiatry and Behavioral Sciences, Stanford School of Medicine, Stanford, California

Disclosure of Interests

The following contributors have indicated that they have no financial interests or other affiliations that represent or could appear to represent a competing interferes with their contributions to this book:

Amy Barnhorst, M.D.; Ana DiRago, Ph.D.; Michael B. Kelly, M.D.; Anne B. McBride, M.D.; Sophie Rosseel, M.D.; Suzanne Shimoyama, M.D.; Kelli Marie Smith, M.D.; Amy Toig, B.A.

Foreword

*We are not here to curse the darkness, but to light the candle that
can guide us through that darkness to a safe and sane future.*

John F. Kennedy

On February 14, 2018, a 19-year-old expelled student walked into Marjory Stoneman Douglas (MSD) High School in Parkland, Florida armed with a legally purchased AR-15 style semiautomatic rifle and multiple magazines. He fired and killed 17 students and staff members and injured 17 others. In 6 short minutes, the United States experienced its deadliest school shooting. Prior to the shooting, the shooter had been assessed by a range of investigators and evaluators, yet interventions to deter him were either not implemented or not successful. Is it possible that an evidence-based assessment or preventative intervention approach might have changed the course of this horrific day?

In the wake of yet another seemingly senseless tragedy, our society is again forced to face three questions that demand effective answers rather than thoughts and prayers alone. First, what are the relevant factors that lead to violence in our schools? Second, how do various disciplines that interact with youth assess potential threats of violence? Third, what interventions have been shown to address and decrease aggression and violence in a school setting?

Safe Passage: A Guide for Addressing School Violence provides practical and effective answers so desperately needed to address the above questions. This outstanding book represents an invaluable resource for psychiatrists, psychologists, social workers, teachers, administrators, judges, probation officers, lawyers, policymakers, and family members, all of whom are architects responsible for constructing a safe passage through the halls of school and the path of a student's life.

This book cogently organizes guidelines for addressing school violence into three parts. The first part consists of seven chapters highly relevant for understanding the foundations of juvenile violence both in and out of the school setting. Among the many topics included in this section, the authors review risk factors for juvenile violence, categories of school violence, limitations on profiling potentially violent youth, bullying and cyberbullying, and factors unique to understanding and addressing youth sexual violence.

The second part provides a state-of-the art review of juvenile threat and violence assessment. The authors provide an excellent summary of threat assessment approaches, a review of the Virginia Model for Student Threat Assessment, specific guidelines on questioning collateral contacts, and developmental considerations when assessing a potentially violent threat. The authors provide an exceptionally easy to understand distillation of commonly used violence risk assessment instruments and assess the utility of such instruments for evaluating threats and potential violence. The authors also address important case law relevant to legal duties to protect third parties from harm. The third and final part reviews interventions important for addressing and decreasing aggression in school and important factors for fostering a healthy school environment.

In each chapter, the authors create a useful learning interface between the reader and the text, which makes this book both engaging and exceptionally practical. The authors assist the reader in understanding potentially complex topics using clearly defined definitions, realistic case vignettes, illustrative diagrams, summary tables, highlighted key points, relevant clinical pearls, and up-to-date epidemiology and relevant references. The editors include three separate appendices that provide example threat assessment questions for use with grade school students, middle school students, and high school and college students. These appendices give structured interview guidelines that serve as an invaluable template for investigating a potentially violent student.

Editors Michael Kelly and Anne McBride have beautifully organized a practical guide for addressing school violence. Echoing the eloquent words of President John F. Kennedy, this book serves to move past cursing the darkness of school violence and instead lighting a candle through that darkness with a safe passage to a sane future.

Charles Scott, M.D.

Preface

School violence is a frightening topic and one that is often equated with mass school shootings. Most Americans today would instantly recognize footage and images from the tragic mass school shooting that occurred on April 20, 1999 at Columbine High School that resulted in the deaths of 12 students, 1 teacher, and the 2 student perpetrators along with the injuries of 21 additional victims. Most individuals who live in the United States hear the words "Virginia Tech" and "Sandy Hook" and immediately visualize mass student casualties after 33 university students and faculty died (and 23 victims were injured) on April 16, 2007 and 20 first-grade students and 6 school personnel were killed at an elementary school on December 14, 2012, respectively. Are school shootings becoming more prevalent? It certainly *feels* that way. At the time of this writing, for example, in 2018, 17 students and school staff were killed and 17 individuals were injured at a high school in Parkland, Florida, on February 14, 2018, and 10 students and teachers were killed with 13 others wounded at a high school in Santa Fe, Texas, on May 18, 2018.

In July 2018, the U.S. Department of Homeland Security posted a grant opportunity for School-Age Trauma Training, offering more than $1.8 million in funding "to establish a long-term, self-sustaining mechanism…to deliver free to the public, lifesaving trauma training to high school age students for mass casualty events" (U.S. Department of Homeland Security 2018). But does our focus on mass casualty events truly address the scope of violence within our schools today? In fact, school violence comes in many different forms, from bullying on campus to trauma off campus to community gangs to violent crimes. Addressing school violence requires a comprehensive and multifaceted approach.

Violence in our schools is an often misunderstood and sensationalized phenomenon. Our hope is that this book appeals to educators, school administrators, mental health clinicians (e.g., psychiatrists, psychologists, social workers), other health care professionals who work with children (e.g., pediatricians, family practice clinicians), and interested laypersons. This book will introduce readers to important concepts pertaining to school violence and serve as a practical guide for mitigating and preventing violence in our schools.

The book is composed of three parts. In Part I, we provide readers with background information on topics that are foundational to performing threat and risk assessments. Important topics covered in this part include the subtyping of aggression, adolescents' proclivity for reward-seeking behaviors, and the development of impulse control. Additional chapters in Part I focus on trauma outside of school, violence on campus, bullying, and sexual violence. We address topic-specific interventions in these chapters as well.

Our understanding of the subtypes of aggression reviewed in Part I forms the basis for threat and risk assessment in Part II. In Part II, we focus on threat assessment and violence risk assessment in a manner that takes individual, school, and community variables into account. Regarding violence risk assessment, every student is evaluated in relation to static risk factors (i.e., historical variables that cannot be changed), dynamic risk factors (i.e., risk factors that are amenable to change), and protective factors. Violence risk is characterized along a continuum rather than in binary fashion. Thus, understanding where a student fits along this spectrum is of utmost importance when identifying opportunities to move the student away from violent behavior. Given that what matters to a third grader is different than what matters to a tenth grader, assessments must be developmentally attuned to individuals. As such, violence risk assessment is a nuanced endeavor considering developmental states as youth progress from elementary school to college.

In Part III, we focus on interventions for preventing, mitigating, and addressing school violence. In this part, we summarize individual and school-based approaches to preventing violence and intervening after violence has occurred. We also provide a methodology for school staff and mental health clinicians to address the school climate itself. Multiple school violence reduction programs are reviewed. This is followed by a brief discussion of the media and its potential influence on our children's perceptions of violence and on their behavior.

As parents, physicians, and educators, we feel strongly that children need safe and supportive environments to learn most effectively. We are both psychiatrists trained in general psychiatry, child and adolescent psychiatry, and forensic psychiatry. Dr. Kelly serves as Senior Psychiatrist at Coalinga State Hospital and Program Director of the Forensic Psychiatry Fellowship at San Mateo County Behavioral Health and Recovery Services. Dr. McBride is the Program Director of the Child and Adolescent Psychiatry Residency at the University of California, Davis. Our educational, scholarly, clinical, and forensic work focuses largely on children and adults who have been disenfranchised through the cumulative effects of poverty, trauma, untreated mental illness, and inadequate access to education. The origins of the problems that plague many of the patients and families we serve begin early in development and can be passed on generationally. It is through such a lens that this text was created.

The editors and authors wish to add that this text has compiled expert perspectives for providing guidance in understanding, assessing, and addressing school violence. Therefore, we cannot accept liability for how this information is applied or for any errors that may exist.

Michael B. Kelly, M.D.
Anne B. McBride, M.D.

Reference

U.S. Department of Homeland Security: School Age Trauma Training (SATT; DHS-ST-108-FR04). Washington, DC, Office of Procurement Operations, Grant Division, July 2018. Available at: www.grants.gov/web/grants/view-opportunity.html?oppId=307563. Accessed August 28, 2018.

Acknowledgments

Thanks to my wife Leah, who makes our family go. This book would not have been possible without your love and support. To my wife, children, their "big sister" Janna, and close friends for making every day a reason to be grateful. To my parents, Brian and Ernestine, my sister Anne, and her husband Andy, for always being in my corner. Also, to my Aunt Bruna Traversaro, whose varied interests inspired my curiosity from an early age. I'd also like to thank the men and women at San Quentin State Prison, with whom I worked while finishing this book. Thank you for helping affirm that this work matters. Despite coming far as a society and advances in the profession, there is still much to be done to ensure that we can all share equitably the freedoms our nation affords. Thanks to my colleagues at Coalinga State Hospital, San Mateo County, and Santa Clara County for the opportunity to continue doing the work that I love. Above all, I'd like to thank God for guidance, whether the road is smooth or rocky.

Michael B. Kelly, M.D.

I dedicate this book to my parents, Helen and Jeff, for giving me the stable childhood that every person deserves. Your lessons in generosity, intellectual curiosity, and sensibility are ones I hope to instill in my own children. To my brave and loving sister, Allison, who first taught me about perseverance and resilience. To my strong and passionate husband, Nick: your support has been unrelenting, and without it I could not do what I do. And most of all, to our three boys—Maximus, Ernest, and Oscar—the inspirations of my life. I am grateful for every moment with each of you. I will strive each day to provide you with the unconditional love, nurturing support, and thoughtful guidance to become exactly the men you are meant to be.

Anne B. McBride, M.D.

PART I
Foundations

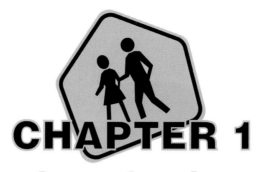

CHAPTER 1

An Introduction to School Violence

Michael B. Kelly, M.D.

Anne B. McBride, M.D.

Arany Uthayakumar, B.A.

Jeff Bostic, M.D., Ed.D.

Sharon Hoover, Ph.D.

Suffering has been stronger than all other teaching, and has taught me to understand what your heart used to be. I have been bent and broken, but—I hope—into a better shape.

Charles Dickens, Great Expectations

Statistically speaking, we live in an age when individuals face the lowest-ever risk of being harmed by others (O'Toole 2000). In fact, overall, youth violence at school has declined in recent decades. For example, the percentage of students in ninth through twelfth grades who reported being threatened or injured with a weapon on school property dropped from 8.4% in 1995 to 6% in 2015 (Centers for Disease Control and Prevention 2017). Additionally, on the basis of the most recent data from the Centers for Disease Control and Prevention, physical fights on school property in the 12 months preceding data collection dropped from roughly 16% in 1993 to 8% in 2015.

Although these data are encouraging, aggression is still a part of everyday life, and violence in our communities is all too common. In the United States, notable disparities exist where the risk of being a victim of violence is concerned. For example, between 1990 and 2010, homicide rates for boys and young men (between 10 and 24 years) who were black or Hispanic were consistently greater than the total homicide rate, whereas homicide rates for white boys and men were lower than the average rate (David-Ferdon et al. 2013). These data underscore the complexities of community violence in the United States.

What drives the continued presence of violence in our youth? From an evolutionary perspective, humans are neurobiologically primed to look out for danger. In fact, humans have more nerve cells attuned to recognizing and recalling negative inputs than positive ones. For much of human history, this predisposition helped keep humans from being blindsided or ambushed by predators and other dangers. In modern society, our species' knack for anticipating and recognizing danger makes us vulnerable to manipulation (Glassner 2010). Media outlets have long known what "makes us tick" and have exploited our predisposition for anxiety to achieve everything from boosting nightly news viewership to selling toothpaste. Given our hardwiring for anxiety, one might assume that contact with violence could serve an adaptive purpose in some way, like a twisted form of exposure therapy. However, exposure to violence does not prepare our children to lead happy lives. In general, being around violence increases our children's vulnerability to negative life experiences and outcomes, including mental illness, physical illness, and reduced psychosocial functioning (Holt et al. 2008; Margolin and Gordis 2000, 2004).

Although exposure to violence can be harmful, aggression is not always problematic. For example, in 1946, while Leo Durocher (manager of the Brooklyn Dodgers baseball team) was preparing for a game against the New York Giants, he was asked by famed sports reporter Red Barber, "Why don't you be a nice guy for a change?" Durocher motioned toward the Giants' dugout and replied, "The nice guys are all over there, in seventh place." Human capacity for aggression is not bad in and of itself. There is actually a growing body of literature defending the potential benefits of adaptive forms of aggression (Banny et al. 2011; Bresin and Gordon 2013; Hawley and Vaughn 2003). A backpacker hiking through the Santa Cruz Mountains, for example, should fight back if attacked by a hungry mountain lion and not play dead. A high school debate team member is likely to perform better when he or she is able to channel aggressive feelings into assertive statements rather than simply agreeing with an opponent. In order to effectively assess and address school violence, we must first identify the type of aggression we are targeting: maladaptive aggression.

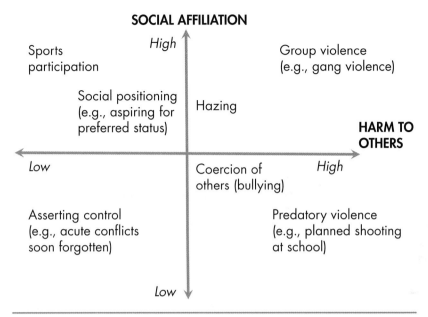

FIGURE 1–1. **Types of school violence: a continuum.**

A Continuum of School Violence

The World Health Organization defines *violence* as "the intentional use of physical force or power, threatened or actual, against oneself, another person, or against a group or community, that either results in or has a high likelihood of resulting in injury, death, psychological harm, maldevelopment, or deprivation" (World Health Organization 2002). This nuanced definition of violence accounts for its potential impacts on the psyche as well as the body. In this text, we offer one simple conceptualization of violence that encompasses traditional interpersonal violence or harm (e.g., assaults, shooting, rape, robbery) as well as social affiliation violence that poses less imminent dangers toward a person yet still involves an exertion of force to the detriment of others for one's own gain or benefit. This conceptualization is depicted in Figure 1–1, which provides axes for categorizing potentially violent events at school.

The two variables just described, *harm* and *social affiliation*, can provide quick clarity for intervention steps. For a student who is high on the axes of both harm and social affiliation, the most apt intervention will not only protect targets but also address the *group* (e.g., the gang, clique, or organization that encourages *hazing*) to alter the group goal of harming those perceived to be interfering with its mission. For a student who is high on the axis of harm but low on the axis of affiliation, the intervention may center on protecting targets and reducing the student's level of isolation from peers. For a student low on axes of both harm and affiliation, the intervention may be focused on conflict resolution and building affiliation for the student (and sometimes also the target). A student who is low on the harm axis and high on the affiliation axis (e.g., captain of the football team) may require an intervention to help him or her become more conscientious about interacting with others while preserving prosocial group affiliations.

In this book, the chapter authors focus on an approach toward integrating our knowledge about maladaptive aggression with the types of violence perpetrated at school. In our view, context is key when attempting to identify, assess, and address maladaptive aggression and school violence. The evidence reveals that comprehensive approaches to addressing school violence are somewhat helpful (Espelage et al. 2013; Evans et al. 2014; Grossman et al. 1997), whereas efforts to profile potential violence perpetrators are minimally helpful (Bailey 2001; O'Toole 2000). For example, screening all students for violent propensities, initially heralded as a mechanism for recognizing and identifying threatening students, resulted in the identification of many students who were not and did not become violent (false positives). At the same time, violent school events (and particularly school shooting massacres) are so rare and difficult to predict that it is challenging to find one assessment tool to predict which student will actually become violent. However, evidence-based risk assessment can help guide the evaluator when working with youth who have been identified as being at risk for perpetrating violence.

Prevention of School Violence
Zero-Tolerance Policies

In addition to attempting to predict perpetrators of violence, much research has focused on general prevention of school violence. We contend, given an abundance of literature, that the zero-tolerance policies enforced at many of our nation's schools are ineffective, despite their good intentions (American Psychological Association Zero Tolerance Task Force 2008; Gregory et al. 2010; Martinez 2009; Skiba and Knesting 2000; Skiba et al. 2011). Literature on adolescent risk taking offers a neurodevelopmental perspective hypothesizing why zero-tolerance policies are ineffective. The dual systems model of adolescent risk taking describes how the growing propensity youth have for reward seeking peaks in adolescence, despite the fact that they are still years away from developing adult-level cognitive control over impulses (Steinberg 2010).

Zero-tolerance policies, discussed in greater depth in Chapter 4, "Danger at Home," do not alter our children's neurobiology, nor are we suggesting that children's neurobiology needs to be changed. In our view, expecting zero-tolerance policies to effectively curb school violence—especially violent acts associated with impulsive aggression—is unrealistic. However, the authors acknowledge that schools have a duty to protect their students from harm, and there has been some legal precedent regarding this duty. For example, in the case of *Rodriguez v. Inglewood Unified School District*, Mr. Rodriguez, a former student at Inglewood High School in southern California, filed a suit against the district because he was stabbed by a nonstudent who had entered the campus (Rodriguez v. Inglewood Unified School District 1986). Mr. Rodriguez claimed that Inglewood High School's previous history of campus violence involving weapons should have prompted the district to institute security measures. In its opinion, the Court of Appeals of California ruled, "A duty is owed by a school district to protect its students by virtue of the special relationship that is created" (p. 723). The Court added that

> the right of all students to a school environment fit for learning cannot be questioned. Attendance is mandatory and the aim of all schools is to teach. Teaching and learning cannot take place without the physical and mental well-being of the students. The school premises, in short, must be safe and welcoming. (p. 715)

This case, and similar cases around the country, underscore the difficulties our educators face in effectively addressing school violence. In our view, the case offers a possible explanation for the motivation behind zero-tolerance policies, despite the existence of strategies that we contend are more effective in general prevention of school violence. We describe those strategies in later chapters.

Developmental Differences

Lawmakers, school district officials, educators, and mental health professionals must be attuned to the significant developmental differences in children. For example, small children often bite and strike each other. As a result, alternative tactics and behaviors are taught and employed in preschools and elementary schools. Adolescents must ultimately attempt to separate from parents and find a place among peers. Therefore, inclusion, exclusion, and intimidation to achieve a preferred status will persist (despite any well-intentioned *no-tolerance* school policies regarding such behaviors) and cross into bullying with repetitive verbal or physical insults toward others. Other adolescents will fear having no place or "home" amid their peers and succumb to gang affiliation over no affiliation to at least feel some semblance of belonging. Accordingly, the interventions for addressing these developmental stages, and the circumstances leading to violence situated within them, become opportunities to address factors contributing to violence within all our communities, starting through our schools. With 15,000 hours of contact and influence on each child from kindergarten through twelfth grade, schools are best positioned to respond to violence and guide students toward more meaningful engagement with others as they approach adulthood.

Conclusion

We cannot eliminate aggression and violence—sports and other human aggressions will outlive all of us. We can, however, seek to redirect a student's violent propensities away from deliberately harming others and toward prosocial pursuits that spare others from harm. Such an approach requires understanding what is driving a student's behavior (e.g., past abuse, peer acceptance, thrill seeking) and the conditions that perpetuate it. At the community level, it behooves us to be mindful of the experiences that may increase our children's propensity for violence (e.g., substance use, trauma, the impact of violent movies and video games) (Anderson et al. 2010; Council on Communications and Media 2009; Prot et al. 2014).

When evaluating the potential for school violence, we assess both students and their environments (e.g., school, home, peer affiliation, community). We focus on risk and protective factors. We seek information that elucidates how to integrate rather than isolate the student. We make efforts to address the circumstances that lead to aggression and violence in a student as early on as possible. We try to prevent or mitigate harm to self, peers, educators, and the community at large. In sum, our text advocates for a comprehensive individualized approach to addressing school violence that prioritizes the consideration of risk factors, the bolstering of protective factors, and the most appropriate treatment for the individual.

Key Points

- In general, being around violence increases our children's vulnerability to negative life experiences and outcomes, including mental illness, physical illness, and reduced psychosocial functioning.

- Comprehensive approaches to addressing school violence are somewhat helpful, whereas efforts to profile potential violence perpetrators are minimally helpful.

- Zero-tolerance policies enforced at many of our nation's schools are ineffective, despite their good intentions.

Clinical Pearls

Understanding school violence on continua involving level of social affiliation and potential for harm can provide a framework for addressing school violence.

Evidence-based risk assessment can help guide the evaluator when working with youth who have been identified as being at risk for perpetrating violence.

When evaluating the potential for school violence, individual students and their environments (e.g., school, home, peer affiliation, community) should be addressed.

References

American Psychological Association Zero Tolerance Task Force: Are zero tolerance policies effective in the schools?: an evidentiary review and recommendations. Am Psychol 63(9):852–862, 2008 19086747

Anderson CA, Shibuya A, Ihori N, et al: Violent video game effects on aggression, empathy, and prosocial behavior in eastern and western countries: a meta-analytic review. Psychol Bull 136(2):151–173, 2010 20192553

Bailey KA: Legal implications of profiling students for violence. Psychol Sch 38(2):141–155, 2001

Banny AM, Heilbron N, Ames A, et al: Relational benefits of relational aggression: adaptive and maladaptive associations with adolescent friendship quality. Dev Psychol 47(4):1153–1166, 2011 21299275

Bresin K, Gordon KH: Aggression as affect regulation: extending catharsis theory to evaluate aggression and experiential anger in the laboratory and daily life. J Soc Clin Psychol 32(4):400–423, 2013

Centers for Disease Control and Prevention: Trends in the Prevalence of Behaviors That Contribute to Violence on School Property. National YRBS: 1991–2015. Atlanta, GA, Centers for Disease Control and Prevention, 2017. Available at: www.cdc.gov/healthyyouth/data/yrbs/pdf/trends/2015_us_violence school_trend_yrbs.pdf. Accessed October 4, 2018.

Council on Communications and Media: From the American Academy of Pediatrics: policy statement—media violence. Pediatrics 124(5):1495–1503, 2009 19841118

David-Ferdon C, Dahlberg LL, Kelger SR: Homicide rates among persons aged 10–24 years—United States, 1981–2010. MMWR Morb Mortal Wkly Rep 62(27):545–548, 2013 23842443

Espelage DL, Low S, Polanin JR, et al: The impact of a middle school program to reduce aggression, victimization, and sexual violence. J Adolesc Health 53(2):180–186, 2013 23643338

Evans CB, Fraser MW, Cotter KL: The effectiveness of school-based bullying prevention programs: a systematic review. Aggress Violent Behav 19(5):532–544, 2014

Glassner B: The Culture of Fear: Why Americans Are Afraid of the Wrong Things. New York, Basic Books, 2010

Gregory A, Cornell D, Fan X, et al: Authoritative school discipline: high school practices associated with lower bullying and victimization. J Educ Psychol 102(2):483–496, 2010

Grossman DC, Neckerman HJ, Koepsell TD, et al: Effectiveness of a violence prevention curriculum among children in elementary school: a randomized controlled trial. JAMA 277(20):1605–1611, 1997 9168290

Hawley PH, Vaughn BE: Aggression and adaptive functioning: the bright side to bad behavior. Merrill-Palmer Q 49(3):239–242, 2003

Holt S, Buckley H, Whelan S: The impact of exposure to domestic violence on children and young people: a review of the literature. Child Abuse Negl 32(8):797–810, 2008 18752848

Margolin G, Gordis EB: The effects of family and community violence on children. Annu Rev Psychol 51(1):445–479, 2000 10751978

Margolin G, Gordis EB: Children's exposure to violence in the family and community. Curr Dir Psychol Sci 13(4):152–155, 2004

Martinez S: A system gone berserk: how are zero-tolerance policies really affecting schools? Prev Sch Fail 53(3):153–158, 2009

O'Toole ME: The School Shooter: A Threat Assessment Perspective. Quantico, VA, Federal Bureau of Investigation Academy, National Center for the Analysis of Violent Crime, Critical Incident Response Group, 2000

Prot S, Gentile DA, Anderson CA, et al: Long-term relations among prosocial-media use, empathy, and prosocial behavior. Psychol Sci 25(2):358–368, 2014 24335350

Rodriguez v. Inglewood Unified School District, 186 Cal. App. 3d 707, 230 Cal. Rptr. 823 (Ct. App. 1986).

Skiba RJ, Knesting K: Zero tolerance, zero evidence: an analysis of school disciplinary practice. New Dir Youth Dev 92:17–43, 2000 12170829

Skiba RJ, Horner RH, Chung C-G, et al: Race is not neutral: a national investigation of African American and Latino disproportionality in school discipline. School Psych Rev 40(1):85–107, 2011

Steinberg L: A dual systems model of adolescent risk-taking. Dev Psychobiol 52(3):216–224, 2010 20213754

World Health Organization: World report on violence and health: summary. Geneva, World Health Organization, 2002

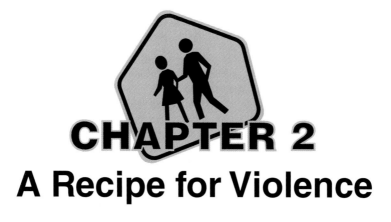

CHAPTER 2
A Recipe for Violence

Immaturity, Impulsivity, and Aggression

Michael B. Kelly, M.D.

Anne B. McBride, M.D.

Jeff Bostic, M.D., Ed.D.

Sharon Hoover, Ph.D.

Ana DiRago, Ph.D.

Arany Uthayakumar, B.A.

The adolescent's mind works differently from ours. Parents know it. This Court has said it. Legislatures have presumed it for decades or more. And now, new scientific evidence sheds light on the differences.

Amici curiae *brief from Roper v. Simmons*

Case Vignette

John and Mike are eighth-grade boys on their school's baseball team. During practice one day, John learns that Mike just began dating John's ex-girlfriend. Mike begins to taunt John, and both boys get into a verbal altercation. Before the head coach can intervene, the verbal altercation quickly escalates into a physical fight. John swings at Mike but misses, and Mike is able to punch John several times before their coaches reach them to break up the fight. John appears humiliated. Once the boys have cooled off, the coaches attempt to talk with them, with the goal of conflict resolution. Mike tells John that he feels terrible for overreacting and fighting his friend. John says little but appears calm. Given that the incident occurred after school on a Friday, a plan is made for the boys to meet with the vice principal on Monday morning. The head coach calls and speaks with Mike's parents about the incident but is unable to reach John's parents because the number on file is no longer in service.

On Monday morning, the school office receives an anonymous tip from a student that John had posted a concerning message on a social media site. Although the message had already been removed, the student reports John had posted "You better watch your back" with a picture of a gun. Mike arrives at the meeting with the vice principal, but John does not attend. In fact, John was absent from his first-period class prior to the scheduled meeting. While the vice principal attempts to contact John's parents, a school monitor spots John around the area of the baseball field. The school resource officer is informed of the situation, and he approaches John. John is initially guarded with the officer but ultimately informs him that he has a plan to harm Mike. John reveals that he has a knife from home in his backpack to carry out his plan.

Violence occurs at school just as it does in every other sphere of life. However, it is important to note that the prevalence of serious violence at schools has, in fact, decreased in recent decades. Data from the U.S. Federal Bureau of Investigation have shown that the number of murders involving a juvenile offender decreased 65% between 1994 and 2003, increased by 32% by 2006, and then decreased by 31% through 2016 (Office of Juvenile Justice and Delinquency Prevention 2018). In fact, students are far more likely to be murdered outside school than while in school. For example, in 1999 alone, for every student killed in a school that year, almost 150 students were killed outside school (Anderson 2001). According to the Youth Risk Behavior Surveys administered nationally to more than 10,000 students each year, there have been declines in physical fighting (16.2% to 7.8%) and weapon carrying (11.8% to 4.1%) at school from 1993 to 2015 (Centers for Disease Control and Prevention 2017). Results from self-report surveys are consistent with other sources of information, indicating a downward trend in juvenile violent crime, including violent crime in schools (Kann et al. 2018).

In this book, the authors propose that educators and clinicians need to understand the individual variables that contribute to a student's aggression and violence in order to address other related problems. Evidence borrowed from literature addressing juvenile delinquency shows that classifying youth only according to the types of offenses committed does little to predict students' likelihood of recidivism or explain why they offended in the first place (Steiner et al. 2001). For instance, knowing that one student physically assaulted another does not tell you why it happened or indicate whether it will happen again.

When planning interventions, there is utility in understanding the subtypes of aggression displayed in relation to the types of violent acts committed (Steiner et al. 2017). In this chapter, we review aggression subtypes and provide an introduction to and brief overview of a range of violent acts that are known to occur at school. Considering the subtypes of aggression displayed, it is critical to remain cognizant of a student's social affiliation and recognize that student's potential for causing serious harm to others.

Aggression Subtypes

Aggression has its place in the mélange of human emotion. Maladaptive aggression is part of that complex parcel. In Dan Connor's (2012) book *Aggression and Antisocial Behavior in Children and Adolescents,* maladaptive aggression is described as 1) aggression occurring outside an expected social context (e.g., a child who beats up a classmate during a church Sunday school lesson), 2) aggressive acts that happen despite the absence of an identifiable trigger (e.g., a grade schooler who "sucker punches" a new student despite never having met before), 3) aggressive behavior that is out of proportion to its antecedent (e.g., a student who flips over his desk and chair after a teacher tells him to put his cell phone away), or 4) aggression that takes a long time to subside (e.g., a high school senior who mercilessly beats up a freshman who bumped him in the hallway and immediately apologizes for the transgression). Such behaviors, especially when presented as a pattern, are a warning sign for underlying psychopathology.

In broad terms, maladaptive aggression can be broken down into planned, instrumental, and predatory (PIP) subtypes versus reactive, affective, defensive, and impulsive (RADI) subtypes (Blair et al. 2010; Padhy et al. 2011; Plattner et al. 2007; Steiner et al. 2003; Vitiello and Stoff 1997) (Table 2–1). Acts of PIP, or "cold," aggression are premeditated and carried out with little remorse or empathy for the victim. The proverb "Revenge is a dish best served cold" succinctly characterizes cold aggression. RADI, or "hot," aggression tends to occur in response to identifiable triggers and is out of proportion to its precipitant. Readers who are familiar with the comic book character the Incredible Hulk may conjure an immediate caricature of hot aggression: the mild-mannered scientist, Bruce Banner, becoming the seething, angry Hulk in response to feeling threatened. Hot and cold aggression have disparate neurodevelopmental underpinnings.

At the neurobiological level, PIP aggression is a form of goal-directed activity that is mediated by the same structures in our brains (e.g., striatum, prefrontal cortex) responsible for all of our goal-directed behaviors (Blair et al. 2006). Thus, acts of PIP aggression tend to be carried out with an anticipated positive outcome in mind. That is, the aggressor plans his or her

TABLE 2–1.   Types of maladaptive aggression

RADI aggression (reactive, affective, defensive, and impulsive)	PIP aggression (planned, instrumental, and predatory)
"Hot" aggression; heat of the moment	"Cold" aggression; calculated
Response to identifiable triggers and often out of proportion to offending incident	Premeditated acts of aggression, little remorse for the victim
Mediated by fight or flight system: connections between paired amygdalae and periaqueductal gray	Mediated by goal-directed structures: striatum, prefrontal cortex
Associated with anxiety disorders, mood disorders, and posttraumatic stress disorder	Associated with callous-unemotional traits, problems recognizing emotions, reduced fight or flight response, and limited remorse

actions, wants to inflict harm, and feels justified in doing so. On an individual level, a propensity for PIP aggression has been associated with problems recognizing emotions in oneself and others, diminished biological reactivity in response to perceived threat (i.e., a reduced "fight or flight" response), and limited remorse. Thus, students with a propensity for PIP aggression may be less inclined to empathize with potential victims while being relatively undeterred by potential consequences. The literature often refers to youth who frequently display this type of aggression as having *callous-unemotional* traits. Such students may be at a higher risk for causing harm, or repeatedly causing harm, to others than are those who tend to engage in more reactive displays of aggression.

RADI aggression, in contrast, has a different neurobiology from the PIP form. RADI is mediated through activation of the fight or flight system, which is largely composed of connections between paired amygdalae in the hippocampi to a portion of the midbrain called the periaqueductal gray (Gregg and Siegel 2001; Panksepp 2004). Unlike the calculating nature of PIP aggression, RADI aggression can be described as occurring in the heat of the moment in response to a perceived threat. It is common for people who engage in reactive forms of aggression to regret their actions once given the opportunity to calm down. RADI aggression has been associated with youth with anxiety disorders, mood disorders, and posttraumatic stress disorder (Ruths and Steiner 2004; Steiner et al. 2011). Although an act of violence can include both types of aggression, it is important to determine whether a youth's actions involve predominantly PIP or RADI aggression, and, to this end, Table 2–2 provides examples of questions to address when a student has committed violence.

TABLE 2–2. **Questions for determining aggression subtypes**

When evaluating a student who has committed an act of violence, the following questions should be addressed:

Was the act of violence premeditated?

Does the student feel empathy or remorse for the victim?

What did the student hope to achieve by committing the act?

What did the student expect the consequences to be?

Aggression can also be described as physical or relational in nature. Physical aggression is easy to identify, but relational aggression can be insidious. We loosely define *relational aggression* as a means of damaging a person's social standing, peer support, and/or self-esteem. Common examples of relational aggression directed at students include verbal bullying, spreading gossip, making verbal threats, and ostracism. Identifying the type of maladaptive aggression a youth has a propensity for (e.g., hot, cold, physical, relational) is fundamental for assessing risk and planning interventions. We discuss relational aggression and associated violence in more detail in Chapter 5, "Bullying and Cyberbullying."

Dual Systems Model of Adolescent Risk-Taking

Literature on adolescent risk-taking yields useful insight into the developmental factors that can exacerbate the challenge of preventing violence in our schools. Laurence Steinberg's (2010) paper "A Dual Systems Model of Adolescent Risk-Taking" examined the hypothesis that adolescents' propensity for risk-taking stems from the differing trajectories of neurobiological systems governing pleasure seeking and impulse control. In other words, the *dual systems model* proposes that young people are biologically primed to engage in reward-seeking behaviors around the time that puberty takes hold; however, their ability to control impulses does not mature until early adulthood.

In order to test his hypothesis, Steinberg studied 935 children and young adults whose reward-seeking behaviors and impulsivity were quantified using both self-reports and behavioral measures (Steinberg 2010). Results showed that reward-seeking behaviors rise rapidly during the preteen years and peak during midadolescence. Although impulse control was shown to steadily improve beginning at age 10, it did so at a relatively slow rate and did not plateau until early adulthood. According to the dual systems model, adolescence is akin to driving a sports car with rapid acceleration and poor brakes. This creates a scenario that predisposes young people to act on their emotions more readily than they ultimately will as adults.

Types of Violence

Violence exists on a continuum. In Chapter 1, "An Introduction to School Violence," we provide clinicians with an axial system for categorizing potentially violent acts at school, which has implications for planning interventions. Benbenishty and Astor (2005) described a socioecological model of school violence that acknowledges the roles that individual, family, school culture, and community factors play in the expression of violence in our schools. Such a perspective is consistent with this book's approach to threat assessment, risk assessment, and intervention.

We define *interpersonal violence* as that which occurs between people when one person intentionally engages in physical (e.g., punching, kicking) or relational (e.g., spreading rumors, cyberbullying, ostracizing) violence against others. A classic example of interpersonal physical violence might be a child who beats up a peer in order to take his or her lunch money. Relational forms of interpersonal violence include intentionally excluding a peer from a group or crafting negative social media posts so as to deliberately hurt a peer's feelings.

A more insidious form of violence also seen in schools is *structural violence*, in which persisting socioeconomic or cultural structures both foment and preserve forces that are conducive to violence. For instance, a youth with absent family support, a history of victimization, and limited financial resources might adapt to his or her situation by turning to a gang for protection and a means of making money (e.g., selling drugs). Such an attempt at leading a better life is understandable if the structures in place within a community (and school) seem to preclude the possibility of success through prosocial endeavors. Thus, structural factors sustaining the potential for violence may predominate over societal maxims that may seem unfruitful to a student on the basis of his or her everyday experience. This discussion is in no way intended to diminish the importance of students taking personal responsibility for their actions. Rather, we contend that in order to help students achieve their full potential and take agency over their lives, an appreciation for the context in which they are raised is paramount. Without recognizing the various structural burdens students may already face, efforts to help will likely prove futile.

Some individuals who have grown up around high levels of interpersonal or structural violence will be resourceful and resilient enough to succeed despite various obstacles. That said, it does not take an extensive background in sociology to understand that interpersonal and structural violence can negatively alter a student's developmental trajectories. An ecological approach to violence includes recognition of personal, school, and community variables that may interfere with a student's trajectory.

Common Manifestations of School Violence

School violence can be categorized into four main types: student conflicts, bullying, gang violence, and mass school shootings. Student conflicts make up the bulk of incidents of school violence. Bullying can significantly alter the school's climate in general and cause significant harm. Gang violence is another manifestation of school violence that can permeate a school, making youth vulnerable to becoming the victims or perpetrators of violence. Mass school shootings, while rare, have catastrophic and lasting effects both on campus and nationwide. Other forms of violence that typically occur off campus (e.g., sexual violence, maltreatment, exposure to domestic violence) can profoundly affect students and schools; these topics are explored in detail in later chapters.

Student Conflicts

The most common form of school violence surrounds isolated conflicts between peers. These conflicts may surround competition, but unlike in bullying, these students do not possess prominent advantages over other students. Rather, two students of similar abilities (e.g., cognitively, physically) may disagree and escalate on a topic. At times, the escalation may involve violent behavior that could be considered a crime (e.g., possession of a weapon on campus, threatening or causing serious harm to classmates or staff). Physical violence on campus is discussed in more detail in Chapter 7, "Growing Up in Fear." For more minor student conflicts, it is impossible for any of us to always emerge victorious from a situation, so learning effective tools for navigating disagreements or resolving differences is essential for all students. These tools will serve them well throughout their lives.

Bullying

Bullying, addressed in more detail in Chapter 5, refers to persistent, distressing efforts by individuals who usually possess more social, verbal, or physical power to intimidate or exert dominance over another. *Social bullying* usually involves people excluding or disparaging, spreading rumors about, or commenting negatively about a peer. The Centers for Disease Control and Prevention (2016) estimate that approximately 20% of students are bullied each year.

According to the National Center for Education Statistics (NCES), when location is specifically identified, bullying occurs most frequently in hallways and stairwells and least often in the bathroom or locker room. Most common forms of bullying are being made fun of, called names, or insulted—reported by approximately 13.3% of students in 2015 (Musu-Gillette et al. 2017). Students reporting being bullied at school declined from 28% in 2005 to 21% in 2015. Girls reported being bullied slightly more than boys.

Today, bullying takes many different forms. More traditional forms of bullying include verbal and physical bullying. *Verbal bullying* includes making hostile, harassing, or threatening comments to a target, whereas *physical bullying* involves imposing unwanted physical contact, pushing, striking, or assaulting a target. Cyberbullying, an increasingly prevalent form of social bullying, continues to rise with children's increased access to the Internet juxtaposed against the limited availability of caretakers to monitor online activity. The 2013 estimates from the NCES indicate that approximately 7% of students reported being cyberbullied anywhere in the past year. (Musu-Gillette et al. 2017). Unwanted contact through texting has been the most common form of cyberbullying (Centers for Disease Control and Prevention 2016).

Bullying peaks in middle school, when students attempt to establish a place among their peers and distinguish the difference between attaining status and "taking" status at the expense of others. A middle schooler's task is to separate from his or her parents and try to find a place among peers. Finding one's status within a peer group is a complex event related to the unique aspirations and expectations of each person in the group. Some peer groups establish a de facto hierarchy easily, with accepted leaders and followers, but many groups experience significant internal pressure from adolescents jockeying for different positions. A possible explanation for this is that, in general, middle school students typically lack sophisticated skills for asserting their aspirations respectfully and have little experience with establishing group hierarchies. It stands to reason that the factors favoring conflict, intimidation, and bullying crescendo during this adolescent task of separating from parents and finding a desirable place among peers.

There are at least four components in most bullying situations.

1. *Perpetrators/bullies* often have a history of having been victimized or bullied themselves.
2. *Targets/victims* of bullying experience pain, humiliation, and ostracism from others, which can ingrain feelings of helplessness and resentment. Students more vulnerable to bullying include those with disabilities (e.g., autism spectrum disorder, learning disabilities, physical disabilities, attention-deficit/hyperactivity disorder, stuttering). Similarly, students perceived to be sexually divergent from

cisgender heterosexual norms are more vulnerable to bullying. Being a bully's target or victim is usually embarrassing for students, so most targets and bystanders/observers do not report incidents of bullying. Impacts of bullying include increased depression, decreased school grades and attendance, and even lowered postsecondary educational aspirations.

3. *Bystanders/observers* do not gain the tools to respond to or alter bullying events from simply observing bullying. Instead, bystanding may cultivate passivity and desensitization if the bystanding itself is not directly addressed. More than 50% of middle schoolers report having been bystanders to bullying (Finley 2014).

4. The *system* of a school, or any organization, can perpetuate bullying behavior. For example, groups (e.g., fraternities, sports teams, musical groups) often tolerate and pass down hazing rituals, which are meant to bring about a sense of community but can devolve into bullying. A different example might include the expectation that a gang member follow gang rules (e.g., targeting another student for violence) at the expense of following school rules. In such situations, unless the status afforded the strongest or most violent student(s) is addressed effectively by school administration, it is unlikely that this type of violence will diminish within that system.

Bullying impacts everyone involved, not just victims and bystanders. For instance, of boys who were classified by researchers as bullies in sixth through ninth grade, approximately 40% were convicted of a crime three or more times by age 24 (Fox et al. 2003). For more detail on the impact of bullying, see Chapter 5.

Gang Violence

Gangs and gang violence in America are almost as old as our nation itself. For instance, many people who immigrated to the United States in the 1800s were fleeing varying degrees of poverty, persecution, and famine. Some were treated as unwelcome guests on arrival in the United States and banded together to form street gangs as a means of forging an identity, obtaining financial gain, and securing political clout. Gangs continue to permeate American culture, and their ranks are often populated with disenfranchised youth. Some of the most significant risk factors for adolescent gang involvement include limited access to education, poor job prospects, a need to belong, and low attachment to the community (Hill et al. 2001; Howell and Egley 2005; Pollard et al. 1999; Wortley and Tanner 2004).

Roughly 20% of students between sixth and twelfth grades report the presence of gangs in their schools (National Center on Addiction and Substance Abuse at Columbia University 2010; Robers et al. 2012 as cited in Howell 2013). Gang involvement alone predisposes young people to problematic substance use, school failure, unemployment, and early parenthood (Krohn et al. 2011 as cited in Simon et al. 2013). Gang-affiliated students are much more likely to be both the perpetrators and victims of violence (National Gang Center 2018). Young people who are in gangs perpetrate far more violent crime while they are in a gang than when they are not in a gang (Howell 2013). Addressing gang violence is discussed in detail in Chapter 7, "Growing Up in Fear," including a description of some programs that can help steer students away from gangs and help them leave gangs if they are currently involved.

Mass School Shootings

School shootings, reviewed in more detail in Chapter 7, are rare yet highly publicized phenomena. As we discuss in Chapter 3, "Inconvenient Truths," profiling school shooters is a tricky, if not impossible, task. However, important lessons have been learned from previous school shootings that are helpful to consider in situations involving a threatened school shooting. The U.S. Secret Service and Department of Education performed a review of 37 targeted school violence incidents occurring between 1974 and 2000 and issued their findings in 2002 (Vossekuil et al. 2002). According to Vossekuil et al. (2002, p. 32), targeted school violence incidents (such as mass shootings) are not random events but instead are the end result of a "comprehensible process of thinking and behavior: behavior that typically began with an idea, progressed to the development of a plan, moved on to securing the means to carry out the plan, and culminated in an attack." For instance, 95% of the attackers studied by Vossekuil and colleagues had been considering their actions for days—sometimes weeks and years—before the attack.

Although the individual victims of school shootings and other attacks may be determined at random, the decision of the person who initiates violence is not random. School shootings are largely predicated on the shooter's relationship with peers, teachers, and the surrounding community. For example, revenge was cited as a motive in 61% of the attacks, and some form of grievance against the victim(s) was identified in 81% of cases (Vossekuil et al. 2002). Interestingly, 93% of attackers engaged in behaviors that in hindsight could have been considered clues (e.g., veiled threats or vague comments pertaining to obtaining and/or using weapons). We discuss this phenomenon, dubbed *leakage*, in greater depth in Chapter 3. We discuss threat assessment, risk assessment, and schoolwide interventions pertaining to student conflicts, bullying, gang violence, and school shootings in Part II, "Threat and Risk Assessment," and Part III, "Interventions."

Key Points

- Maladaptive aggression can be categorized as one of two subtypes: 1) planned, instrumental, and predatory (PIP, or "cold" aggression) or 2) reactive, affective, defensive, and impulsive (RADI, or "hot" aggression). Both types of aggression differ in their neurobiological underpinnings, social origins, and associated disorders.

- The dual systems model of adolescent risk-taking posits that the contradictory tendency to seek out risk despite not having developed impulse control arises from the divergence of pathways in the brain overseeing these processes. In other words, neurobiological hardwiring leads youth to engage in risky behaviors, although their impulse control will not mature until adulthood.

- Violence exists as a spectrum, and in this chapter we have examined the definitions of interpersonal and structural violence on this continuum. Understanding structural violence, and the socioeconomic and cultural factors that precede it, will be pivotal in enacting effective interventions.

Clinical Pearls

Students who commit premeditated violent acts and feel no remorse (PIP aggression) are at a higher risk for repeatedly causing harm than are students who engage in a violent act in response to a perceived threat (RADI aggression).

RADI aggression can be described as occurring in the heat of the moment in response to a perceived threat. RADI aggression has been associated with youth with anxiety disorders, mood disorders, and posttraumatic stress disorder.

When trying to understand why a student committed certain acts, consider how these behaviors fit within the student's socioeconomic and cultural structure. Behaviors that may be adaptive in specific structures can be maladaptive in other contexts, such as school.

References

Anderson RN: Deaths: leading causes for 1999. Natl Vital Stat Rep 49(11):1–87, 2001 11682979

Benbenishty R, Astor RA: School Violence in Context: Culture, Neighborhood, Family, School, and Gender. New York, Oxford University Press, 2005

Blair RJ, Peschardt KS, Budhani S, et al: The development of psychopathy. J Child Psychol Psychiatry 47(3–4):262–276, 2006 16492259

Blair RJR, Niranjan SK, Coccaro EF, et al: Taxonomy and neurobiology of aggression, in Principles and Practice of Child and Adolescent Forensic Mental Health. Edited by Benedek EP, Ash P, Scott CL. Washington, DC, American Psychiatric Publishing, 2010, pp 267–278

Centers for Disease Control and Prevention: Understanding School Violence. Atlanta, GA, Centers for Disease Control and Prevention, 2016. Available at: www.cdc.gov/violenceprevention/pdf/school_violence_fact_sheet-a.pdf. Accessed October 4, 2018.

Centers for Disease Control and Prevention: Trends in the Prevalence of Behaviors That Contribute to Violence on School Property. National YRBS: 1991–2015. Atlanta, GA, Centers for Disease Control and Prevention, 2017. Available at: www.cdc.gov/healthyyouth/data/yrbs/pdf/trends/2015_us_violence school_trend_yrbs.pdf. Accessed October 4, 2018.

Connor DF: Aggression and Antisocial Behavior in Children and Adolescents: Research and Treatment. New York, Guilford, 2012

Finley LL: School Violence: A Reference Handbook. Boston, MA, ABC-CLIO, 2014

Fox JA, Elliott DS, Kerlikowske RG, et al: Bullying Prevention Is Crime Prevention. Washington, DC, Fight Crime: Invest in Kids, 2003

Gregg TR, Siegel A: Brain structures and neurotransmitters regulating aggression in cats: implications for human aggression. Prog Neuropsychopharmacol Biol Psychiatry 25(1):91–140, 2001 11263761

Hill KG, Lui C, David Hawkins J: Early Precursors of Gang Membership: A Study of Seattle Youth. Washington, DC, U.S. Department of Justice, Office of Justice Programs, Office of Juvenile Justice and Delinquency Prevention, 2001

Howell JC: Why is gang-membership prevention important? Changing Course: Preventing Gang Membership. Edited by Simon TR, Ritter NM, Mahendra RR. Washington, DC, National Institute of Justice, 2013, pp 7–18

Howell JC, Egley A Jr: Moving risk factors into developmental theories of gang membership. Youth Violence Juv Justice 3(4):334–354, 2005

Kann L, McManus T, Harris WA, et al: Youth Risk Behavior Surveillance—United States, 2017. MMWR Surveill Summ 67(8):1–114, 2018 29902162

Krohn MD, Ward JT, Thornberry TP, et al: The cascading effects of adolescent gang involvement across the life course. Criminology 49(4):991–1028, 2011

Musu-Gillette L, Zhang A, Wang K, et al: Indicators of School Crime and Safety: 2016 (NCES 2017-064/NCJ 250650). Washington, DC, National Center for Education Statistics and Bureau of Justice Statistics, 2017

National Center on Addiction and Substance Abuse at Columbia University: National Survey of American Attitudes on Substance Abuse XV: Teens and Parents, 2010. New York, National Center on Addiction and Substance Abuse at Columbia University, 2010

National Gang Center: Frequently Asked Questions About Gangs. Washington, DC, National Gang Center, 2018. Available at www.nationalgangcenter.gov. Accessed October 6, 2018.

Office of Juvenile Justice and Delinquency Prevention: OJJDP Statistical Briefing Book. Washington, DC, Office of Juvenile Justice and Delinquency Prevention, 2018. Available at: www.ojjdp.gov/ojstatbb/offenders/qa03105.asp?qaDate =2016. Accessed April 3, 2019.

Padhy R, Saxena K, Remsing L, et al: Symptomatic response to divalproex in subtypes of conduct disorder. Child Psychiatry Hum Dev 42(5):584–593, 2011 21706221

Panksepp J: Affective Neuroscience: The Foundations of Human and Animal Emotions. New York, Oxford University Press, 2004

Plattner B, Karnik N, Jo B, et al: State and trait emotions in delinquent adolescents. Child Psychiatry Hum Dev 38(2):155–169, 2007 17417724

Pollard JA, Hawkins JD, Arthur MW: Risk and protection: are both necessary to understand diverse behavioral outcomes in adolescence? Soc Work Res 23(3):145–158, 1999

Robers S, Zhang J, Truman J: Indicators of School Crime and Safety: 2011 (NCES 2012–002/NCJ 236021). National Center for Education Statistics. Washington, DC, U.S. Department of Justice, Office of Justice Programs, Bureau of Justice Statistics, and U.S. Department of Education, 2012

Ruths S, Steiner H: Psychopharmacologic treatment of aggression in children and adolescents. Pediatr Ann 33(5):318–327, 2004 15162638

Simon TR, Ritter NM, Mahendra RR: Changing Course: Preventing Gang Membership. Washington, DC, National Institute of Justice, 2013

Steinberg L: A dual systems model of adolescent risk-taking. Dev Psychobiol 52(3):216–224, 2010 20213754

Steiner H, Humphreys K, Redlich A: The Assessment of the Mental Health System of the California Youth Authority: Report to Governor Gray Davis. Stanford, CA, Stanford University, 2001

Steiner H, Saxena K, Chang K: Psychopharmacologic strategies for the treatment of aggression in juveniles. CNS Spectr 8(4):298–308, 2003 12679744

Steiner H, Silverman M, Karnik NS, et al: Psychopathology, trauma and delinquency: subtypes of aggression and their relevance for understanding young offenders. Child Adolesc Psychiatry Ment Health 5(1):21, 2011 21714905

Steiner H, Daniels W, Stadler C, et al: Disruptive Behavior: Development, Psychopathology, Crime, and Treatment. New York, Oxford University Press, 2017

Vitiello B, Stoff DM: Subtypes of aggression and their relevance to child psychiatry. J Am Acad Child Adolesc Psychiatry 36(3):307–315, 1997 9055510

Vossekuil B, Fein R, Reddy M, et al: The Final Report and Findings of the Safe School Initiative: Implications for the Prevention of School Attacks in the United States. Washington, DC, U.S. Department of Education, Office of Elementary and Secondary Education, Safe and Drug-Free Schools Program and U.S. Secret Service, National Threat Assessment Center, 2002

Wortley S, Tanner J: Social groups or criminal organizations? The extent and nature of youth gang activity in Toronto, in From Enforcement and Prevention to Civic Engagement: Research on Community Safety. Toronto, ON, Canada, University of Toronto Centre of Criminology, 2004, pp 59–80

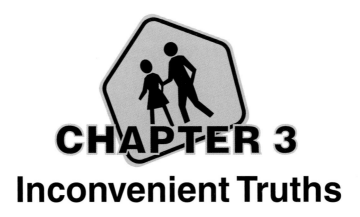

CHAPTER 3
Inconvenient Truths

Profiling and Its Limitations

Anne B. McBride, M.D.

Michael B. Kelly, M.D.

Ana DiRago, Ph.D.

Amy Toig, B.A.

Arany Uthayakumar, B.A.

Prediction is difficult, especially when dealing with the future.

Danish proverb

Case Vignette

Tyler is a 14-year-old freshman with a history of fights with peers, argumentativeness toward teachers, defiance, and multiple school absences. He has an Individualized Education Program for a specific learning disability (reading and writing) and receives services for speech and language impairment. Earlier in the school year, Tyler confided in one of his teachers that the bruises on his arms resulted from a fight with his mother's boyfriend. Tyler's teacher subsequently reported the incident to Child Protective Services. Tyler steals marijuana from his mother's boyfriend and smokes it daily after school.

During lunch, two students begin fighting. Tyler jumps in and begins to punch one of the students. He does not stop punching the student until school security physically restrains him. Tyler screams to the other student that he is going to kill him next time and pantomimes shooting him with a gun.

Attempts by law enforcement agencies to create reliable profiles for criminal offenders date back to the 1970s and 1980s (Groth et al. 1977; Hazelwood 1987). However, there is no evidence to support the existence of distinct criminal profiles (Goodwill et al. 2009; Snook et al. 2008). From a developmental psychopathology perspective, there is limited value to classifying students according to the types of violent acts or crimes they have committed for the purpose of creating profiles (Steiner et al. 2001).

By 2002, the U.S. Secret Service (O'Toole 2009) and the Federal Bureau of Investigation (FBI) and U.S. Department of Education (Vossekuil et al. 2002) concluded that it is more harmful than helpful to profile students suspected of posing a threat to school. There are very few students who ultimately act out such threats when compared with the number of students who may have characteristics consistent with a profile, and the labeling and surveillance of those identified students would both be unjustified and likely inaccurate. Instead, both agencies recommended that schools respond to all threats quickly and fairly with a threat assessment approach to impede acts of school violence. Threats are defined as occurring when a person threatens to commit an act of violence or engages in threatening behavior or targeted violence. Threat assessment should be applied to students who *pose* a threat, even if the student did not verbalize or formally make a threat to others (Cornell 2018).

Profiling lacks the necessary sensitivity and specificity to be considered a reliable tool in the prevention of violence. The current literature suggests that when attempting to understand the root causes of violent behavior, focusing on personal, family, peer, and community variables is more important than considering profiles or diagnostic labels (Steiner et al. 2017). Thus, it is dubious to categorize youth on the basis of the type of crime committed without considering their developmental levels and unique histories. Although juvenile offenders cannot be neatly profiled by criminal typology, examining subtypes of offenders yields certain trends that may affect treatment and general outcomes.

General Violence

Youth violence rates vary depending on how they are measured. Data from the FBI in 2015 indicated that juveniles younger than 18 years accounted for 10.2% of all violent crime arrests, which included 605 arrests for murder, 2,745 arrests for forcible rape, and 21,993 arrests for aggravated assault (Federal Bureau of Investigation 2015). However, these arrest rates do not necessarily represent the extent of youth violence. For example, in the National Youth Risk Behavior Survey of nearly 15,000 youth between ninth and twelfth grades, 23.6% of youth reported being in a physical fight in the 12 months prior to the survey, 15.7% reported carrying a weapon on one or more of the preceding 30 days, and 4.8% reported carrying a gun on at least one day during the preceding 12 months (Kann et al. 2018).

There is no single profile of the typical juvenile violent offender. This being said, it can be useful to distinguish between various pathways to violent behavior and to understand general trends related to trajectories of youth offenders. As described in Chapter 2, "A Recipe for Violence," violence in general is often characterized as either reactive (reactive, affective, defensive, and impulsive [RADI], "hot") or proactive (planned, instrumental, and predatory [PIP], "cold") aggression. *Reactive aggression* is generally thought to be more impulsive, motivated by anger, and retaliatory in response to provocation, whether real or perceived. *Proactive aggression* refers to more predatory violence—often unprovoked, deliberate or planned, and generally goal-directed. When evaluating youth violence, understanding this basic distinction between types of violence and the distinct etiologies involved is key to determining the most effective course of treatment. For example, a youth who commits mostly reactive aggression may respond better to treatment that includes anger management, whereas a youth engaging in only proactive aggression may require intensive management that includes therapies geared toward improving empathy for others.

Understanding general trajectories of youth violent offenders is also important. In general, delinquent and violent behavior peaks in adolescence. Despite the relative peak in violence, most youth who are violent or aggressive do not continue to engage in these behaviors into adulthood. Moffitt (1993) was one of the first researchers to propose two main trajectories of juvenile offenders, distinguishing between a small group of youth engaging in antisocial behavior throughout every stage of life (life-course-persistent antisocial behavior) and a large group of youth who engage in antisocial behaviors only during adolescence (adolescent-limited antisocial behavior). The etiologies of the two subtypes were thought to be distinct, with the early and persistent offenders' behavior relating to the combination of neuropsychological variation with poor environmental factors and the transient offenders' behaviors relating more to almost normative delinquent behavior emerging during a high-risk maturity gap.

Moffitt's ideas were later refined on the basis of research on the male members of the Dunedin Multidisciplinary Health and Development Study in New Zealand. This study followed youth from age 3 to age 26 (Moffitt et al. 2002). Through this work, Moffitt and colleagues identified four main groups of males (Table 3–1). The majority were either abstainers, who did not engage in delinquency or criminal behaviors, or

TABLE 3–1. Groups identified from the Dunedin Multidisciplinary Health and Development Study

Abstainers	Chronic, low-level offenders	Adolescent-limited offenders	Life-course-persistent offenders
Did not engage in delinquency	Demonstrated internalized issues, such as anxiety and depression	Demonstrated increased mental health problems and substance dependency and committed offenses (e.g., property-related crimes)	Demonstrated more extreme psychopathic personality traits and mental health problems and engaged in more drug-related and violent crime

chronic but low-level offenders, who exhibited more internalizing problems (e.g., anxiety, depression, social isolation). Moffitt et al. (2002) found a continued distinction between the adolescent-limited offenders and the life-course-persistent offenders. At age 26, the adolescent-limited offenders still presented with elevated impulsive personality traits, mental health problems, substance dependence, financial problems, and property offenses. The life-course-persistent offenders were more extreme at age 26 and, of the four groups, were most elevated on psychopathic personality traits; mental health problems; substance dependence; number of children; financial problems; work problems; and drug-related and violent crime, including violence against women and children. The life-course-persistent offenders accounted for 10% of the study participants.

In the Pathways to Desistance study (Steinberg et al. 2015), researchers examined the trajectories of 1,354 youth offenders in Arizona and Pennsylvania over 7 years. Their sample included mostly youth ages 14–18 years who had been adjudicated delinquent or found guilty of one or more serious violent crimes, property offenses, or drug offenses (no more than 15% of male drug offenders were included). Of the study's participants, the index event was the first petition to court for 25.5% of the offenders, and 69% had two or more petitions to court before the index petition. More than 40% of participants had been adjudicated of felony crimes against persons (i.e., murder, robbery, aggravated assault, sex offense, and kidnapping). The youth were interviewed repeatedly over time, and information was verified through collateral interviews with a family member or friend and a review of official records.

After 7 years, the study identified five group trajectories (Figure 3–1): 37.2% of participants were offending at a low rate consistently throughout

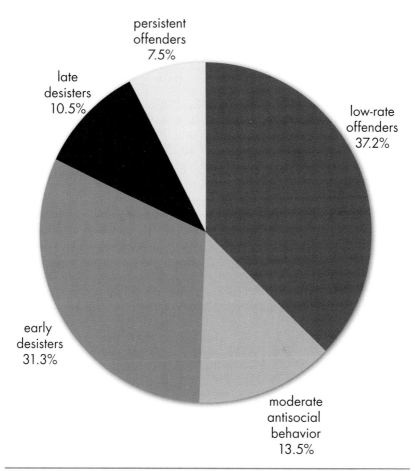

FIGURE 3–1. Group trajectories identified from the Pathways to Desistance Study.

the time period; 13.5% of participants consistently exhibited moderate antisocial behavior; 31.3% of participants were early desisters, exhibiting high offending early, followed by steady and rapid decline in such behavior during early adolescence; 10.5% of participants were late desisters, participating in high rates of antisocial behavior through midadolescence, peaking at age 15, followed by decline through to adulthood; and 7.5% of participants were persistent offenders, consistently displaying high levels of offending between ages 14 and 25 years. The authors concluded that most juvenile offending is limited to adolescence and that the vast majority of juvenile offenders desist from engaging in antisocial behaviors as they transition to adulthood. Notably, desistance occurred even in youth who committed serious crimes.

Furthermore, the authors also identified an association between levels of psychosocial maturity (e.g., ability to control impulses, consider implications of actions for others, delay gratification, or resist peer influence) and engagement in criminal behaviors. They observed that youth whose antisocial behavior persisted into early adulthood displayed lower levels of psychosocial maturity in adolescence and deficits in their development of maturity overall, suggesting that general maturation is associated with maturing out of participation in criminal behavior. Interestingly, the authors found that psychosocial maturation continued at age 25, albeit at a slower rate, and that individuals from all antisocial trajectory groups exhibited higher levels of general psychosocial maturity over time (Steinberg et al. 2015).

Juvenile Sexual Violence

Presently, juvenile sexual violence, discussed in greater depth in Chapter 6, "Understanding and Addressing Youth Sexual Violence," is a research area of interest within the field of school violence. Broadly, *sexual violence* can be defined as a sexual act that is committed or attempted by another person without freely given consent of the victim or against someone who is unable to consent or refuse. It includes forced or alcohol- or drug-facilitated penetration of a victim; forced or alcohol- or drug-facilitated incidents in which the victim is made to penetrate a perpetrator or someone else; nonphysically pressured unwanted penetration; intentional sexual touching; or noncontact acts of a sexual nature. Sexual violence can also occur when a perpetrator forces or coerces a victim to engage in sexual acts with a third party (Basile et al. 2014). Estimates of sexual offending in general suggest that male adolescents perpetrate 20% of all rapes and 30%–50% of child molestation and that youth younger than age 20 are responsible for approximately 50% of sexually aggressive incidents in the United States (Shaw and Antia 2010). A large body of research indicates that juvenile sex offenders constitute a heterogeneous group of youth offenders rather than a unique profile of individuals. Moreover, this research asserts that most juvenile sex offenders do not continue to engage in sexual offending into adulthood—a finding that is in line with research examining youth violence in general. Overall, when compared with adult sex offenders, juvenile sex offenders appear more similar as a group to nonsexual-offending juvenile delinquents (Ryan and Otonichar 2016).

Ryan and Otonichar (2016) reported that juvenile sex offenders have been generally classified into three subtypes: youth with paraphilic disorders, youth with conduct disorders, and youth with more general psychopathology. These authors further noted that most juvenile sex offenders do not go on to develop paraphilic disorders. However, as reported by Abel et al. (1985), in adults with paraphilic disorders, 42%

reported development of deviant sexual interests by age 15, and 57% reported development of deviant sexual interests by age 19, suggesting that early intervention for this subgroup is especially important.

Shaw and Antia (2010) identified four types of general sex offenders, noting that juvenile sex offenders tend to combine various features of each group. They identified offenders with true paraphilias, antisocial youth who engaged in sexual offending as part of a larger conduct problem, juveniles with psychiatric or neurobiological disorders impairing impulse regulation, and socially and interpersonally impaired or delayed youth seeking sexual gratification from younger children given lack of an available or appropriate peer group.

Many of the risk factors that apply to sexually aggressive youth apply to juvenile violence offenders in general. There is a wide range of prevalence of sexual victimization in the juvenile offender's own history depending on the study examined, but research has shown that most sexual abuse victims do not grow up to engage in sexual abuse against others. Empirically supported risk factors for male juvenile sexual reoffending specifically include deviant sexual interests, having numerous past sexual offenses, and offending against a stranger (Ryan 2016). Notably, recidivism for sexual offending by juveniles is low (5%–15%) when offenders are treated (Shaw and Antia 2010), although the low recidivism may also be consistent with general trajectories of juvenile sex offenders as described earlier.

Despite the lack of a unique profile of "typical" juvenile sex offenders, research has drawn attention to a subset of youth who engage in sexual offending alone. For instance, a meta-analysis by Pullman and Seto (2012) showed that most adolescent sex offenders can be considered generalists, rather than specialists, in regard to the types of violent acts they perform. The subset of adolescent sex offenders in their analysis who were specialists (i.e., had a history of committing only sexual offenses) tended to have a personal history of childhood abuse and unusual sexual interests. Another study conducted in Singapore involving 156 boys with a history of sexual offending looked at the variety of crimes committed and the boys' rates of recidivism. The boys who had committed sexual offenses alone (i.e., no additional types of crimes) were more likely to sexually offend against their family members than were adolescents who had displayed more criminal versatility (Chu and Thomas 2010). These studies hint that there may be a distinct developmental pathway associated with becoming a specialist juvenile sexual offender, although more research in this area is needed.

School Shooters

The topic of school shooters is explored in further detail in Chapter 7, "Growing Up in Fear." The stereotype of the isolated, brooding, poorly

found that the violence rate was 31%. The most common stalking methods included physical approach, telephone calls, and letter writing.

Purcell and colleagues published a study of 299 Australian juveniles (ages 9–18 years) who engaged in stalking behaviors (Purcell et al. 2009). Their sample population came from a search of court records of consecutive applications for restraining orders, and they defined stalking as the reporting of multiple unwanted intrusions that persisted for more than 2 weeks. They found that the majority, or 64%, of perpetrators were male, and most were high schoolers with a mean age of 15.4 years. The study was limited because its data collection methods relied indirectly on victim statements to determine rates of substance misuse and mental illness, which were low. However, the authors noted that only one case had been referred for psychiatric evaluation. Sixty-nine percent of victims were female, and, notably, 57% of cases involved same-gender stalking.

With regard to the relationship between the perpetrator and victim, Purcell and colleagues found that 98% of victims knew the perpetrator, with only 2% of victims reporting being stalked by a stranger (Purcell et al. 2009). These relationships were noted as shown in Figure 3–2.

Reported behaviors included unwanted approaches, telephone calls, text messaging, and being followed. Regarding rates of violent behaviors, 75% of victims reported being threatened, and 15% of victims reported threats made against a secondary target, such as a relative or friend. Fifty-four percent of victims reported being assaulted in the form of kicking, scratching, or punching. In several cases, victims reported sustaining head injuries or losing consciousness from strangulation, and five victims reported surviving serious sexual assaults.

The authors were able to classify the juvenile stalking behaviors on the basis of six broad categories motivating the behaviors. These categories were stalking as an extension of bullying (28%), retaliating stalkers (individuals motivated by retaliation for some perceived injury or slight, 22%), rejected stalkers following intimate or dating relationships (22%), disorganized and disturbed stalkers with no clear precipitant other than general chronic conduct problems (20%), predatory stalkers (those whose goal is to impose unwanted sexual contact on the victim, 5%), and intimacy-seeking stalkers (2%). Notably, predatory stalkers had the highest rate of assault, including sexual assault, when compared with all other categories of juvenile stalkers.

Purcell et al. (2009) summarized that stalking behavior in juveniles is distinct from adult stalking, particularly given the significantly higher rate of threats and violence observed in juveniles. Additionally, female perpetrators were more frequently observed in juvenile stalking, and the use of accomplices was more prevalent. Motivation for juvenile stalking appeared to differ significantly from that of the adult population; in juveniles, stalking as an extension of bullying was the most

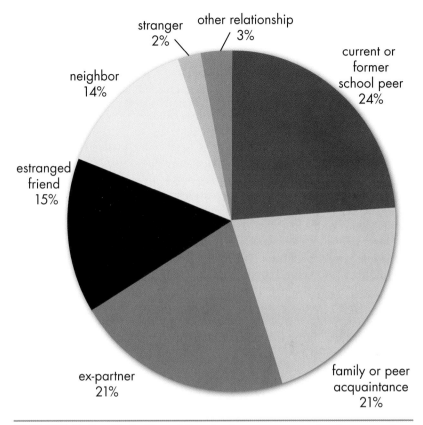

FIGURE 3–2. Relationships between perpetrators and victims.

Source. Adapted from Purcell et al. 2009.

prevalent, whereas stalking related to infatuation or the imposition of an unwanted relationship was extremely uncommon.

Although treatment varies per individual engaging in juvenile stalking behaviors, in general, it is essential to minimize contact between the stalker and victim. When juvenile stalking extends to the school grounds, school and security staff should be educated regarding the behaviors and the need to prevent contact between the perpetrator and victim. In some cases, obtaining a restraining order or filing official charges is warranted.

Case Vignette *(continued)*

Tyler is escorted to the vice principal's office and says that he jumped into the fight to defend another freshman who was being beaten up by a much larger junior. Tyler says that he hates bullies and begins to cry. School administrators notify the police, who ultimately go to Tyler's home because of concerns about access to firearms. The police conclude that Tyler does not have access to firearms. School administrators consider whether Tyler's assaultive behavior and pantomimed gesture are grounds for expulsion. The principal refers Tyler for a mental health evaluation. The mental health professional recommends intensive support services, including individual and family therapy. Tyler returns to the school following a brief suspension.

Key Points

- Profiling is generally ineffective.

- Most juvenile delinquency, violence, and maladaptive aggression do not continue into adulthood.

- Juvenile sex offenders share more similarities with juvenile delinquents who are not sex offenders than with adults who fall in the sex offender category.

- Juvenile stalking behaviors are distinct from adult stalking behaviors, with different motivations and notably higher rates of threats and violence.

Clinical Pearls

Persons planning acts of violence will sometime engage in *leakage* (i.e., intentionally or unintentionally revealing clues regarding impending violence).

Educating students about violence risk factors and fostering a school culture where students "look out" for each other is a practical strategy for preventing campus violence.

In the juvenile population, stalking is more commonly an extension of bullying.

References

Abel GG, Mittleman MS, Becker JV: Sex offenders: results of assessment and recommendations for treatment, in Clinical Criminology: The Assessment and Treatment of Criminal Behaviour. Edited by BenAron H, Hucker S, Wevster C. Toronto, ON, Canada, M&M Graphics, 1985, pp 191–205

Basile KC, Smith SG, Breiding MJ, et al: Sexual Violence Surveillance: Uniform Definitions and Recommended Data Elements, Version 2.0. Atlanta, GA, National Center for Injury Prevention and Control, Centers for Disease Control and Prevention, 2014

Chu CM, Thomas SD: Adolescent sexual offenders: the relationship between typology and recidivism. Sex Abuse 22(2):218–233, 2010 20458125

Cornell D: Comprehensive School Threat Assessment Guidelines: Intervention and Support to Prevent Violence. Charlottesville, VA, School Threat Assessment Consultants, 2018

Federal Bureau of Investigation: Crime in the United States, 2015. Uniform Crime Reports. Washington, DC, U.S. Department of Justice, 2015. Available at: https://ucr.fbi.gov/crime-in-the-u.s/2015/crime-in-the-u.s.-2015. Accessed August 2017.

Goodwill AM, Alison LJ, Beech AR: What works in offender profiling? A comparison of typological, thematic, and multivariate models. Behav Sci Law 27(4):507–529, 2009 19437553

Groth AN, Burgess W, Holmstrom LL: Rape: power, anger, and sexuality. Am J Psychiatry 134(11):1239–1243, 1977 910975

Hazelwood RR: Analyzing the rape and profiling the offender, in Practical Aspects of Rape Investigation: A Multidisciplinary Approach. Edited by Hazelwood RR, Burgess AW. Boca Raton, FL, CRC Press, 1987, pp 169–199

Kann L, McManus T, Harris WA, et al: Youth Risk Behavior Surveillance—United States, 2017. MMWR Surveill Summ 67(SS-08):1–171, 2018 29902162

McCann JT: A descriptive study of child and adolescent obsessional followers. J Forensic Sci 45(1):195–199, 2000 10641939

Moffitt TE: Adolescence-limited and life-course-persistent antisocial behavior: a developmental taxonomy. Psychol Rev 100(4):674–701, 1993 8255953

Moffitt TE, Caspi A, Harrington H, et al: Males on the life-course-persistent and adolescence-limited antisocial pathways: follow-up at age 26 years. Dev Psychopathol 14(1):179–207, 2002 11893092

O'Toole ME: The School Shooter: A Threat Assessment Perspective. Quantico, VA, National Center for the Analysis of Violent Crime, Federal Bureau of Investigation, 2000

O'Toole ME: The School Shooter: A Threat Assessment Perspective. Collingdale, PA, Diane Publishing, 2009

Pullman L, Seto MC: Assessment and treatment of adolescent sexual offenders: implications of recent research on generalist versus specialist explanations. Child Abuse Negl 36(3):203–209, 2012 22445287

Purcell R, Moller B, Flower T, et al: Stalking among juveniles. Br J Psychiatry 194(5):451–455, 2009 19407277

Ryan EP: Juvenile sex offenders. Child Adolesc Psychiatr Clin N Am 25(1):81–97, 2016 26593121

Ryan EP, Otonichar JM: Juvenile sex offenders. Curr Psychiatry Rep 18(7):67, 2016 27222141

Shaw JA, Antia DK: Sexually aggressive youth, in Principles and Practice of Child and Adolescent Forensic Mental Health. Edited by Benedek E, Ash P, Scott C. Washington, DC, American Psychiatric Publishing, 2010, pp 389–402

Snook B, Cullen RM, Bennell C, et al: The criminal profiling illusion: what's behind the smoke and mirrors? Crim Justice Behav 35(10):1257–1276, 2008

Steinberg LD, Cauffman E, Monahan K: Psychosocial Maturity and Desistance From Crime in a Sample of Serious Juvenile Offenders. Laurel, MD, U.S. Department of Justice, Office of Justice Programs, Office of Juvenile Justice and Delinquency Prevention, 2015

Steiner H, Humphreys K, Redlich A: The Assessment of the Mental Health System of the California Youth Authority: Report to Governor Gray Davis. Stanford, CA, Stanford University, 2001

Steiner H, Daniels W, Stadler C, et al: Disruptive Behavior: Development, Psychopathology, Crime, and Treatment. New York, Oxford University Press, 2017

Vossekuil B, Fein R, Reddy M, et al: The Final Report and Findings of the Safe School Initiative: Implications for the Prevention of School Attacks in the United States. Washington, DC, U.S. Department of Education, Office of Elementary and Secondary Education, Safe and Drug-Free Schools Program and U.S. Secret Service, National Threat Assessment Center, 2002

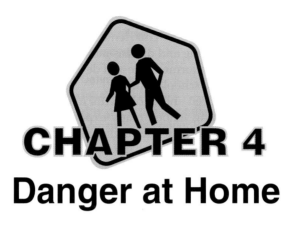

CHAPTER 4
Danger at Home

Addressing Violence Outside School

Suzanne Shimoyama, M.D.

Marcia Unger, M.D, M.P.H.

Suzanne Shimoyama, M.D.
Marcia Unger, M.D, M.P.H.

Safety and security don't just happen; they are the result of collective consensus and public investment. We owe our children, the most vulnerable citizens in our society, a life free of violence and fear.

Nelson Mandela

Case Vignette

Joe is an 8-year-old second grader attending a public elementary school. He lives in an apartment with his mother and her boyfriend (not his father). Although he performed well in first grade, Joe has struggled academically in second grade. He requires frequent reminders to stay on task in class, and on the playground, he is excessively controlling with his peers. Joe has anger outbursts when the game is not going his way. When Joe swears at and pushes his classmate, his teacher takes him to the principal's office. In her office, the principal notices bruises on Joe's neck and arm in the shape of an adult's handprint. Because she is a mandated reporter, the principal contacts Child Welfare to report suspected child maltreatment.

In this chapter, we describe patterns of violence outside school, including experienced and witnessed violence. We present an overview

TABLE 4–1.   **Definitions of terms related to child maltreatment** *(continued)*

Term	Definition
Parental substance abuse	Prenatal exposure of a child to harm due to the mother's use of an illegal drug or other substance; manufacture of a controlled substance in the presence of a child or on the premises occupied by a child; allowing a child to be present where the chemicals or equipment for the manufacture of controlled substances are used or stored; selling, distributing, or giving drugs or alcohol to a child; or use of a controlled substance by a caregiver that impairs the caregiver's ability to adequately care for the child. Some states include parental substance abuse in their definition of abuse and neglect.
Abandonment	Occurs when the parent's identity or whereabouts are unknown, the child has been left by the parent in circumstances in which the child suffers serious harm, or the parent has failed to maintain contact with the child or to provide reasonable support for a specified period of time. Nearly one-third of states include abandonment in their definition of abuse or neglect.

Note.   The definitions of "child" and "child abuse and neglect" are defined by the Child Abuse Prevention and Treatment Act (P.L. 111-320). All other definitions are described by the Child Welfare Information Gateway.

analysis of risk factors for child maltreatment, Brown et al. (1998) identified the existence of multiple risk factors that span multiple domains, from the individual level (child or adult characteristics) to the macrosystem or sociocultural context. They also found that different risk factors may be associated with varying types of abuse. For example, early separation from the mother, perinatal problems, and low maternal involvement are risk factors for physical abuse; poverty and large family size are risk factors for neglect; and female gender, disability, having a deceased parent, and living with a stepfather are risk factors for sexual abuse. Furthermore, Brown and colleagues found several risk factors associated with multiple forms of maltreatment. For instance, factors associated with a higher risk of both childhood physical abuse and neglect include early separation from the mother, low paternal involvement, low paternal warmth, low maternal education, poor marital quality, maternal dissatisfaction with the child, serious maternal illness, and welfare dependency. Maternal sociopathy and young maternal age are risk factors for physical abuse, sexual abuse, and neglect. Brown et al. (1998) also found a relationship between the number of risk factors present and the likelihood of experiencing abuse or neglect: the prevalence of abuse or neglect was 3% with no risk factors and 24% with four or more risk factors identified.

Other studies have shown that boys tend to experience physical abuse slightly more frequently than do girls, and adolescents are more likely than children of other ages to be injured (Finkelhor et al. 2013). However, infants and toddlers are at the highest risk of severe abuse and represent the largest percentage of fatalities as a result of abuse (Child Welfare Information Gateway 2014).

According to a 2018 U.S. Department of Health and Human Services report, the majority (91.4%) of perpetrators of child abuse were one of the victim's parents (Children's Bureau 2018). Child care providers, foster parents, legal guardians, and friends or neighbors each made up 1% or less of the perpetrators. Other perpetrators included 6.2% other relatives; 3.6% unmarried partners of parents and "other," which included foster siblings, nonrelatives, and household staff; and 3.8% clergy. According to the U.S. Department of Health and Human Services Child Welfare Outcomes report, in 2014 the number of children who experienced maltreatment while in foster care varied from state to state, with an overall average of 0.25% (Child Welfare Information Gateway 2014).

Mandating Reporting

In 1974, the United States enacted federal legislation to address child abuse and neglect. The Child Abuse Prevention and Treatment Act (CAPTA) provides federal funding and guidance to states for the establishment of agencies tasked with child abuse prevention, assessment, investigation, prosecution, and treatment. This agency is known as Child Protective Services in many states, but its title may vary from state to state. CAPTA provides an overall definition for abuse and neglect; however, civil and criminal statues may vary from state to state. Standards for reporting may also differ slightly from state to state; however, all 50 states have mandated reporting laws. Some standards require the reporter to have knowledge of conditions that could reasonably result in harm to a child, whereas others simply require a suspicion or reason to believe a child has been a victim of maltreatment.

Maltreatment may include physical abuse, sexual abuse, prenatal drug exposure, neglect, and exposure to intimate partner violence (Mathews and Kenny 2008). As of 2019, mandated reporters of child abuse and neglect include individuals who generally have contact with children (Child Welfare Information Gateway, U.S. Department of Health and Human Services, www.childwelfare.gov). They may include teachers and other school staff; mental health professionals, including counselors and psychiatrists; social workers, health care workers, including physicians and nurses; law enforcement officers; and child care providers. In Delaware, Florida, Idaho, Indiana, Kentucky, Maryland, Mississippi, Nebraska, New Hampshire, New Jersey, New Mexico, North Carolina, Oklahoma, Rhode Island, Tennessee, Texas, Utah, and Wyoming, any person who is suspicious of child abuse or neglect, regardless of profession, is required to report it to child welfare authorities. Suspected abuse is believed to be underreported for a variety of reasons, which may include fear of consequences if a report turns out to be unsubstantiated. However, all states provide some measure of protection for good-faith reporting, and failure to report suspected abuse may lead to lawsuits, criminal charges, and loss of licensing (Schilling and Zolotor 2018).

In 2016, the greatest percentage of child welfare reports were made by education personnel (18.9%), followed closely by legal and law enforcement personnel (18.4%), and then social services personnel (11.2%), medical personnel (9.5%), relatives (6.8%), parents (6.6%), mental health personnel (5.9%), friends and neighbors (4.2%), child care providers (0.6%), alleged victims (0.5%), foster care providers (0.4%), and alleged perpetrators (0.1%). "Other," anonymous sources, and unknown sources make up the remaining 17.1% (Children's Bureau 2018). The fact that school personnel make up the largest group of reporters of abuse underscores the important, even if unintended, role our schools play in the identification of children experiencing abuse and neglect.

Case Vignette *(continued)*

Joe is now 15 years old and a freshman in high school. He has an Individualized Education Program for emotional disturbance due to his history of trauma and problematic behaviors in the classroom. The previous year, he was removed from his biological mother's home because of abuse and neglect and placed in foster care. Joe recently transferred to a trauma-sensitive school after he was expelled from two other high schools in his school district following multiple suspensions for fighting. During class one day, Joe was talking to a peer about a school project. Joe became agitated for reasons unknown to the teacher and started yelling, "I'm going to kill you!" to his classmate. Everyone in the class became frightened, and Joe was escorted out of the room by staff.

Trauma Symptoms

Children exposed to interpersonal violence or who are victims of violence may express this trauma in a variety of ways. Trauma symptoms may be characterized as internalizing or externalizing (Figure 4–1).

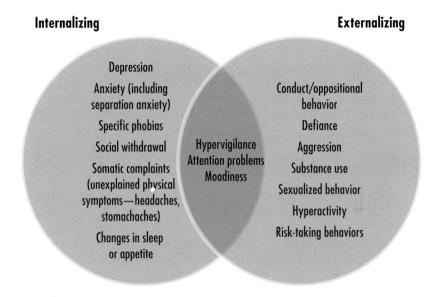

Internalizing   **Externalizing**

Depression

Anxiety (including separation anxiety)

Specific phobias

Social withdrawal

Somatic complaints (unexplained physical symptoms—headaches, stomachaches)

Changes in sleep or appetite

Hypervigilance
Attention problems
Moodiness

Conduct/oppositional behavior

Defiance

Aggression

Substance use

Sexualized behavior

Hyperactivity

Risk-taking behaviors

FIGURE 4–1. **Trauma symptoms.**

Symptoms described as *internalizing* are typically directed inward and may include depression, anxiety, and social withdrawal. *Externalizing* symptoms may include oppositional behavior, aggression, hyperactivity, hypersexualized behavior, and substance use (Gauthier-Duchesne et al. 2017).

A 1998 study by Jane Knapp found that infants who were exposed to domestic violence may exhibit disrupted sleep, poor feeding, excessive screaming, and delayed achievement of developmental milestones (Knapp 1998). Additionally, preschoolers who witness domestic violence tend to have more anxiety, social withdrawal, and nightmares and may show signs of regression such as bedwetting after previously being toilet trained. Trauma symptoms of school-age children vary greatly; however, a decline in school performance may be an important indicator of a child's inner turmoil. Previously well-behaved children may appear more emotionally unstable or get into fights at school. Children exposed to trauma may also complain of somatic symptoms such as stomachaches or headaches. Adolescents tend to exhibit more externalizing symptoms, such as rebelliousness, drug use, running away, and rage.

Because trauma symptoms are heterogeneous, recognizing them in children and adolescents in school settings and without the aid of a screening tool may be challenging. Emotional dysregulation and behavioral changes may be the first clues teachers and school staff notice in children who have experienced trauma. These may occur following a trigger, or reminder of the trauma. For example, a teacher raising his voice to command the attention of an unruly class might trigger a strong emotional response in a child who is reminded of his abuser. Other clues that a student may be experiencing sequelae of trauma or violence include avoidance, social withdrawal, significant changes in friend groups, and self-injurious behaviors. Finally, when a young child is observed with sexualized behaviors, a history of sexual abuse must be considered (Cohen et al. 2016).

Impact of Trauma

A child's exposure to violence, whether witnessed or experienced, can have both immediate and lasting effects. Several studies have shown that childhood maltreatment leads to worse outcomes in terms of physical health and socioeconomic status. Exposure to violence can also cause acute functional impairment and lead to long-term mental health consequences (Roberts et al. 2010). Different types of abuse may have differing but lasting effects on children's behavior (Ford et al. 2011). Multiple studies have shown that mere exposure to interpersonal violence (IPV), not just being a victim of violence, affects a significant portion of children. A 2009 study by Graham-Bermann and colleagues looked at 219 children ages 6–12 years who were exposed to IPV. Using cluster analysis, separating the children into relatively homogeneous groups, the researchers found that nearly a quarter of the sample had severe internalizing and externalizing problems; 45% were struggling, with low global self-worth and social competence scores; 11% were depressed; and the remaining 20% were resilient, with no significant problems reported (Graham-Bermann et al. 2009). School-age children (6–12 years old) who experience IPV may have difficulties developing and maintaining friendships and may have higher levels of conflict with peers. They may exhibit mood swings, anxiety, or social withdrawal (Lundy and Grossman 2005). Graham-Bermann and Levendosky (1998) found that more than half of children who had witnessed IPV exhibited intrusive thoughts (unwelcome involuntary thoughts that are distressing or disturbing) about the exposure, 42% reported symptoms of hyperarousal (a state of increased psychological and physiological tension that may include an exaggerated startle response), and 13% met full criteria for posttraumatic stress disorder (Box 4–1).

Box 4–1.   DSM-5 Diagnostic Criteria for Posttraumatic Stress Disorder

---

Posttraumatic Stress Disorder

Note: The following criteria apply to adults, adolescents, and children older than 6 years. For children 6 years and younger, see corresponding criteria below.

A. Exposure to actual or threatened death, serious injury, or sexual violence in one (or more) of the following ways:

1. Directly experiencing the traumatic event(s).
2. Witnessing, in person, the event(s) as it occurred to others.
3. Learning that the traumatic event(s) occurred to a close family member or close friend. In cases of actual or threatened death of a family member or friend, the event(s) must have been violent or accidental.
4. Experiencing repeated or extreme exposure to aversive details of the traumatic event(s) (e.g., first responders collecting human remains; police officers repeatedly exposed to details of child abuse).

   Note: Criterion A4 does not apply to exposure through electronic media, television, movies, or pictures, unless this exposure is work related.

B. Presence of one (or more) of the following intrusion symptoms associated with the traumatic event(s), beginning after the traumatic event(s) occurred:

1. Recurrent, involuntary, and intrusive distressing memories of the traumatic event(s).

   Note: In children older than 6 years, repetitive play may occur in which themes or aspects of the traumatic event(s) are expressed.
2. Recurrent distressing dreams in which the content and/or affect of the dream are related to the traumatic event(s).

   Note: In children, there may be frightening dreams without recognizable content.
3. Dissociative reactions (e.g., flashbacks) in which the individual feels or acts as if the traumatic event(s) were recurring. (Such reactions may occur on a continuum, with the most extreme expression being a complete loss of awareness of present surroundings.)

   Note: In children, trauma-specific reenactment may occur in play.
4. Intense or prolonged psychological distress at exposure to internal or external cues that symbolize or resemble an aspect of the traumatic event(s).
5. Marked physiological reactions to internal or external cues that symbolize or resemble an aspect of the traumatic event(s).

C. Persistent avoidance of stimuli associated with the traumatic event(s), beginning after the traumatic event(s) occurred, as evidenced by one or both of the following:

1. Avoidance of or efforts to avoid distressing memories, thoughts, or feelings about or closely associated with the traumatic event(s).
2. Avoidance of or efforts to avoid external reminders (people, places, conversations, activities, objects, situations) that arouse distressing memories, thoughts, or feelings about or closely associated with the traumatic event(s).

D. Negative alterations in cognitions and mood associated with the traumatic event(s), beginning or worsening after the traumatic event(s) occurred, as evidenced by two (or more) of the following:

1. Inability to remember an important aspect of the traumatic event(s) (typically due to dissociative amnesia and not to other factors such as head injury, alcohol, or drugs).
2. Persistent and exaggerated negative beliefs or expectations about oneself, others, or the world (e.g., "I am bad," "No one can be trusted," "The world is completely dangerous," "My whole nervous system is permanently ruined").
3. Persistent, distorted cognitions about the cause or consequences of the traumatic event(s) that lead the individual to blame himself/herself or others.
4. Persistent negative emotional state (e.g., fear, horror, anger, guilt, or shame).
5. Markedly diminished interest or participation in significant activities.
6. Feelings of detachment or estrangement from others.
7. Persistent inability to experience positive emotions (e.g., inability to experience happiness, satisfaction, or loving feelings).

E. Marked alterations in arousal and reactivity associated with the traumatic event(s), beginning or worsening after the traumatic event(s) occurred, as evidenced by two (or more) of the following:

1. Irritable behavior and angry outbursts (with little or no provocation) typically expressed as verbal or physical aggression toward people or objects.
2. Reckless or self-destructive behavior.
3. Hypervigilance.
4. Exaggerated startle response.
5. Problems with concentration.
6. Sleep disturbance (e.g., difficulty falling or staying asleep or restless sleep).

F. Duration of the disturbance (Criteria B, C, D, and E) is more than 1 month.

G. The disturbance causes clinically significant distress or impairment in social, occupational, or other important areas of functioning.

H. The disturbance is not attributable to the physiological effects of a substance (e.g., medication, alcohol) or another medical condition.

Specify whether:

With dissociative symptoms: The individual's symptoms meet the criteria for posttraumatic stress disorder, and in addition, in response to the stressor, the individual experiences persistent or recurrent symptoms of either of the following:

1. **Depersonalization:** Persistent or recurrent experiences of feeling detached from, and as if one were an outside observer of, one's mental processes or body (e.g., feeling as though one were in a dream; feeling a sense of unreality of self or body or of time moving slowly).
2. **Derealization:** Persistent or recurrent experiences of unreality of surroundings (e.g., the world around the individual is experienced as unreal, dreamlike, distant, or distorted).

Note: To use this subtype, the dissociative symptoms must not be attributable to the physiological effects of a substance (e.g., blackouts, behavior during alcohol intoxication) or another medical condition (e.g., complex partial seizures).

Specify if:

With delayed expression: If the full diagnostic criteria are not met until at least 6 months after the event (although the onset and expression of some symptoms may be immediate).

Posttraumatic Stress Disorder for Children 6 Years and Younger

A. In children 6 years and younger, exposure to actual or threatened death, serious injury, or sexual violence in one (or more) of the following ways:

1. Directly experiencing the traumatic event(s).
2. Witnessing, in person, the event(s) as it occurred to others, especially primary caregivers.

   Note: Witnessing does not include events that are witnessed only in electronic media, television, movies, or pictures.

3. Learning that the traumatic event(s) occurred to a parent or caregiving figure.

B. Presence of one (or more) of the following intrusion symptoms associated with the traumatic event(s), beginning after the traumatic event(s) occurred:

1. Recurrent, involuntary, and intrusive distressing memories of the traumatic event(s).

   Note: Spontaneous and intrusive memories may not necessarily appear distressing and may be expressed as play reenactment.

2. Recurrent distressing dreams in which the content and/or affect of the dream are related to the traumatic event(s).

   Note: It may not be possible to ascertain that the frightening content is related to the traumatic event.

3. Dissociative reactions (e.g., flashbacks) in which the child feels or acts as if the traumatic event(s) were recurring. (Such reactions may occur on a continuum, with the most extreme expression being a complete loss of awareness of present surroundings.) Such trauma-specific reenactment may occur in play.
4. Intense or prolonged psychological distress at exposure to internal or external cues that symbolize or resemble an aspect of the traumatic event(s).
5. Marked physiological reactions to reminders of the traumatic event(s).

C. One (or more) of the following symptoms, representing either persistent avoidance of stimuli associated with the traumatic event(s) or negative alterations in cognitions and mood associated with the traumatic event(s), must be present, beginning after the event(s) or worsening after the event(s):

Persistent Avoidance of Stimuli

1. Avoidance of or efforts to avoid activities, places, or physical reminders that arouse recollections of the traumatic event(s).
2. Avoidance of or efforts to avoid people, conversations, or interpersonal situations that arouse recollections of the traumatic event(s).

Negative Alterations in Cognitions

3. Substantially increased frequency of negative emotional states (e.g., fear, guilt, sadness, shame, confusion).
4. Markedly diminished interest or participation in significant activities, including constriction of play.
5. Socially withdrawn behavior.
6. Persistent reduction in expression of positive emotions.

D. Alterations in arousal and reactivity associated with the traumatic event(s), beginning or worsening after the traumatic event(s) occurred, as evidenced by two (or more) of the following:

1. Irritable behavior and angry outbursts (with little or no provocation) typically expressed as verbal or physical aggression toward people or objects (including extreme temper tantrums).
2. Hypervigilance.
3. Exaggerated startle response.
4. Problems with concentration.
5. Sleep disturbance (e.g., difficulty falling or staying asleep or restless sleep).

E. The duration of the disturbance is more than 1 month.
F. The disturbance causes clinically significant distress or impairment in relationships with parents, siblings, peers, or other caregivers or with school behavior.
G. The disturbance is not attributable to the physiological effects of a substance (e.g., medication or alcohol) or another medical condition.

Specify whether:

With dissociative symptoms: The individual's symptoms meet the criteria for posttraumatic stress disorder, and the individual experiences persistent or recurrent symptoms of either of the following:

1. **Depersonalization:** Persistent or recurrent experiences of feeling detached from, and as if one were an outside observer of, one's mental processes or body (e.g., feeling as though one were in a dream; feeling a sense of unreality of self or body or of time moving slowly).

2. **Derealization:** Persistent or recurrent experiences of unreality of surroundings (e.g., the world around the individual is experienced as unreal, dreamlike, distant, or distorted).

Note: To use this subtype, the dissociative symptoms must not be attributable to the physiological effects of a substance (e.g., blackouts) or another medical condition (e.g., complex partial seizures).

Specify if:

With delayed expression: If the full diagnostic criteria are not met until at least 6 months after the event (although the onset and expression of some symptoms may be immediate).

A 2002 study by Lansford and colleagues showed that children who experienced physical maltreatment in the first 5 years of life were at risk for psychological and behavioral problems that persisted into adolescence and over the 12-year duration of the study (Lansford et al. 2002). These problems, including posttraumatic stress symptoms, thought difficulties, social problems, social withdrawal, anxiety, depression, dissociation, and aggression, were rated higher than those of their nonmaltreated peers. Child maltreatment can also contribute to criminal behavior. A 1989 study by C.S. Widom found a statistically significant increase in frequency of violent offenses, property offenses, and sex offenses in abused or neglected males compared with control subjects (Widom 1989).

The Centers for Disease Control and Prevention–Kaiser Permanente Adverse Childhood Experiences Study (Centers for Disease Control and Prevention 2014), conducted from 1995 to 1997, included the collection of data from more than 17,000 adults regarding their childhood experiences and current health status and behaviors. This survey included questions about adverse childhood experiences (ACEs), including childhood exposure to various types of abuse, household challenges such as household substance abuse and parental separation or divorce, and emotional or physical neglect (Table 4–2). The results revealed that almost two-thirds of study participants reported at least one ACE, and more than one in five reported three or more ACEs. Furthermore, the study showed a relationship between an increased number of ACEs and negative health and well-being outcomes throughout a person's life (Felitti et al. 1998). Examples of these negative health and well-being outcomes include alcoholism, fetal death, depression, liver and heart disease, poor academic achievement, suicide attempts, and unintended pregnancies.

The Adverse Childhood Experiences Study demonstrated that children who have experienced ACEs are not only at increased risk for disease and early death but also social, emotional, and cognitive impairments. A recent study by Blodgett and Lanigan (2018) also showed that children who have three or more ACEs were three times more likely to experience academic failures. Fifty-two percent of students with three or more ACEs experienced multiple school problems, compared with only 12% of students with no known ACEs (Blodgett and Lanigan 2018). Children with three or more ACEs were also five times more likely to have attendance issues and six times more likely to exhibit behavioral problems (Sporleder and Forbes 2016).

Case Vignette *(continued)*

Joe goes to the school's "calm room" after he leaves the classroom. After the class is dismissed, his teacher goes to the calm room to discuss the incident with Joe. While processing the incident with his teacher, Joe describes how frustrated he is that his foster mother cannot afford to buy him the supplies necessary to complete his school project. He says that he just "lost it" and felt that the other student was intentionally targeting him, knowing that he was feeling overwhelmed and had a short fuse. The teacher, taking a trauma-sensitive approach, gives Joe an in-school suspension rather than a traditional out-of-school suspension. Joe is able to complete his school project by using the materials supplied by the school during his in-school suspension time and successfully passes his freshman year without any further incidents.

Trauma-Informed or Trauma-Sensitive Schools

A trauma-informed or trauma-sensitive school is a school where staff have specific training and education about how trauma affects children in all areas of their life, including education. These schools not only are designed with academic achievement in mind but also consider a child's emotional and physical well-being. A trauma-informed program approaches an individual holistically. The goal of this type of program is to decrease the risk of retraumatization while also providing an environment to aid in recovery from traumatic stress (Sporleder and Forbes 2016).

TABLE 4–2. Adverse Childhood Experiences Study questions on childhood exposure to abuse and household dysfunction

Adverse childhood experience	Questions
Childhood exposure to abuse	

Psychological abuse	Did a parent or other adult in the household
	    often or very often swear at you, insult you, or put you down?
	    often or very often act in a way that made you afraid that you would be physically hurt?

Physical abuse	Did a parent or other adult in the household
	    often or very often push, grab, shove, or slap you?
	    often or very often hit you so hard that you had marks or were injured?

Sexual abuse	Did an adult or person at least 5 years older ever
	    touch or fondle you in a sexual way?
	    have you touch their body in a sexual way?
	    attempt oral, anal, or vaginal intercourse with you?
	    actually have oral, anal, or vaginal intercourse with you?

Household dysfunction	
Substance abuse	Did you ever live with anyone who was a problem drinker or alcoholic? Did you ever live with anyone who used street drugs?
Mental illness	Was a household member depressed or mentally ill? Did a household member attempt suicide?

Mother treated violently	Was your mother (or stepmother)
	    sometimes, often, or very often pushed, grabbed, or slapped or had something thrown at her?
	    sometimes, often, or very often kicked, bitten, hit with a fist, or hit with something hard?
	    ever repeatedly hit over at least a few minutes?
	    ever threatened with, or hurt by, a knife or gun?

Criminal behavior in household	Did a household member go to prison?

Source. Centers for Disease Control and Prevention 2014.

Collectively, these well-intentioned policies and practices can undermine feelings of safety for students impacted by trauma and inadvertently contribute to a school climate counter to many principles of a trauma-informed approach (National Child Traumatic Stress Network Schools Committee 2017). Being in school is considered a protective factor against delinquent behavior (U.S. Department of Health and Human Services 2001); suspending and removing students from school increases the risk of delinquent behaviors. School connectedness is linked to regular school attendance, high graduation rates, and improved academics (Teske 2011).

Neuroscience research has shown that specific structures in the brain are less well developed in adolescents than in adults. Adolescents are more likely to take greater risks and to reason less adequately about the consequences of their behavior (American Psychological Association Zero Tolerance Task Force 2008). Although maintaining school safety is a paramount concern, reliance on zero-tolerance policies exclusively may exacerbate the challenges facing the disciplined youth and the school as a whole.

Implementation of Trauma-Informed Care

The Substance Abuse and Mental Health Services Administration (SAMHSA) has defined a trauma-informed approach as

> A program, organization, or system that is a trauma-informed: 1) realizes the widespread impact of trauma and understands potential paths for recovery; 2) recognizes the signs and symptoms of trauma in clients, families, staff and others involved with the system; 3) responds by fully integrating knowledge about trauma into policies, procedures and practices; 4) seeks to actively resist re-traumatization. (SAMHSA's Trauma and Justice Strategic Initiative 2014, p. 9)

SAMHSA further outlines six key principles of a trauma-informed setting: safety; trustworthiness and transparency; peer support; collaboration and mutuality; empowerment; and gender, cultural and historical issues (Figure 4–2).

The most important aspect of creating a trauma-informed or trauma-sensitive school is the need for a whole-school approach. It is not necessary to screen all children for traumatic experiences, which runs the risk of further stigmatizing those who have encountered trauma in their lives. An effective approach is to ensure that the entire school provides a trauma-sensitive learning environment for all children. Everyone (e.g., administrators, educators, paraprofessionals, par-

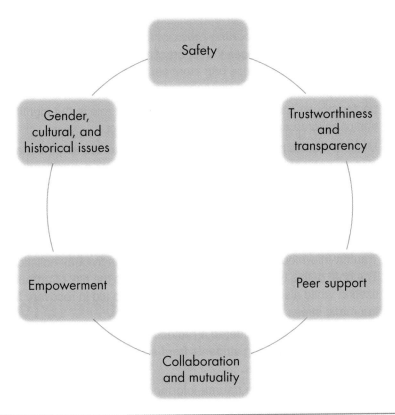

FIGURE 4–2. **Substance Abuse and Mental Health Services Administration (SAMHSA) principles of a trauma-informed setting.**

ents, custodians, bus drivers, lunch personnel) must be part of the schoolwide team to ensure a trauma-sensitive school (Cole et al. 2005).

Key Points

- Exposure to violence is pervasive and most commonly occurs in the home. Children's response to this trauma is not uniform and may manifest in a number of ways, both obvious and subtle, and may result in social and academic difficulties at school.

- Exposure to violence has a lasting impact. Symptoms may be present immediately following the violent exposure and often continue to impact the child into adolescence and adulthood.

Christian CW, American Academy of Pediatrics Committee on Child Abuse and Neglect: The evaluation of suspected child physical abuse. Pediatrics 135(5):e1337–e1354, 2015 25917988

Cohen JA, Mannarino AP, Deblinger E: Treating Trauma and Traumatic Grief in Children and Adolescents. New York, Guilford, 2016

Cole SF, O'Brien JG, Gadd MG, et al: Helping Traumatized Children Learn: Supportive School Environments for Children Traumatized by Family Violence. Boston, Massachusetts Advocates for Children, 2005

Felitti VJ, Anda RF, Nordenberg D, et al: Relationship of childhood abuse and household dysfunction to many of the leading causes of death in adults: the Adverse Childhood Experiences (ACE) Study. Am J Prev Med 14(4):245–258, 1998 9635069

Finkelhor D: Children's Exposure to Violence: A Comprehensive National Survey. Collingdale, PA, Diane Publishing, 2009

Finkelhor D, Turner HA, Shattuck A, et al: Violence, crime, and abuse exposure in a national sample of children and youth: an update. JAMA Pediatr 167(7):614–621, 2013 23700186

Finkelhor D, Turner H, Hamby SL, et al: Polyvictimization: Children's Exposure to Multiple Types of Violence, Crime, and Abuse: National Survey of Children's Exposure to Violence. Washington, DC, Office of Justice Programs, 2011

Ford JD, Gagnon K, Connor DF, et al: History of interpersonal violence, abuse, and nonvictimization trauma and severity of psychiatric symptoms among children in outpatient psychiatric treatment. J Interpers Violence 26(16):3316–3337, 2011 21362676

Gauthier-Duchesne A, Hébert M, Daspe MÈ: Gender as a predictor of posttraumatic stress symptoms and externalizing behavior problems in sexually abused children. Child Abuse Negl 64:79–88, 2017 28040616

Graham-Bermann SA, Levendosky AA: Traumatic stress symptoms in children of battered women. J Interpers Violence 13(1):111–128, 1998

Graham-Bermann SA, Gruber G, Howell KH, et al: Factors discriminating among profiles of resilience and psychopathology in children exposed to intimate partner violence (IPV). Child Abuse Negl 33(9):648–660, 2009 19804905

Howell KH, Barnes SE, Miller LE, et al: Developmental variations in the impact of intimate partner violence exposure during childhood. J Inj Violence Res 8(1):43–57, 2016 26804945

Knapp JF: The impact of children witnessing violence. Pediatr Clin North Am 45(2):355–364, 1998 9568015

Lansford JE, Dodge KA, Pettit GS, et al: A 12-year prospective study of the long-term effects of early child physical maltreatment on psychological, behavioral, and academic problems in adolescence. Arch Pediatr Adolesc Med 156(8):824–830, 2002 12144375

Lundy M, Grossman SF: The mental health and service needs of young children exposed to domestic violence: supportive data. Fam Soc 86(1):17–29, 2005

Mathews B, Kenny MC: Mandatory reporting legislation in the United States, Canada, and Australia: a cross-jurisdictional review of key features, differences, and issues. Child Maltreat 13(1):50–63, 2008 18174348

National Child Traumatic Stress Network Schools Committee: Creating, Supporting, and Sustaining Trauma-Informed Schools: A System Framework. Los Angeles, CA, National Center for Child Traumatic Stress, 2017

Roberts AL, Gilman SE, Fitzmaurice G, et al: Witness of intimate partner violence in childhood and perpetration of intimate partner violence in adulthood. Epidemiology 21(6):809–818, 2010 20811285

Schilling S, Zolotor AJ: Domestic violence, abuse, and neglect, in Chronic Illness Care. Berlin, Germany, Springer, 2018, pp 121–132

SAMHSA's Trauma and Justice Strategic Initiative: SAMHSA's Concept of Trauma and Guidance for a Trauma-Informed Approach. Rockville, MD, Substance Abuse and Mental Health Services Administration, July 2014

Sporleder J, Forbes H: The Trauma-Informed School: A Step-by-Step Implementation Guide for Administrators and School Personnel. Boulder, CO, Beyond Consequences Institute, 2016

Teske SC: A study of zero tolerance policies in schools: a multi-integrated systems approach to improve outcomes for adolescents. J Child Adolesc Psychiatr Nurs 24(2):88–97, 2011 21501285

U.S. Department of Health and Human Services: Youth Violence: A Report of the Surgeon General. Washington, DC, U.S. Department of Health and Human Services, 2001

Widom CS: Child abuse, neglect, and violent criminal behavior. Criminology 27(2):251–271, 1989

Zolkoski SM, Bullock LM: Resilience in children and youth: a review. Child Youth Serv Rev 34(12):2295–2303, 2012

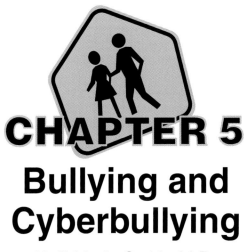

CHAPTER 5
Bullying and Cyberbullying

Kelli Marie Smith, M.D.

Michael B. Kelly, M.D.

My pain may be the reason for somebody's laugh.
But my laugh must never be the reason for somebody's pain.

Charlie Chaplin

Case Vignette

Lana is an 11-year-old girl sent to a psychiatric crisis center after reporting suicidal thoughts to her school counselor. She recently moved to the area and started sixth grade 2 weeks ago. Lana informs her counselor that she has become the target of a bullying campaign on social media and group texts from classmates. The popular girls have been making fun of Lana at school and started a group text thread that they use to spread rumors about her with the rest of the school. The girls started posting digitally altered images of Lana with exaggerated facial features and the word "Llama" above them via group text and social media sites. Lana is most upset by false rumors that she is sexually active with multiple boys at school. Lana explains to her counselor how things are especially difficult at school because everyone believes the girls. Lana wants to "just disappear" and "make it all go away." She has begun to stay home from school and has stopped talking to her parents.

Historically, the relationship between bullying and serious health consequences garnered limited public attention. In fact, school bullying was often accepted as a normative experience of childhood and adolescence and even a rite of passage into adulthood (Arseneault et al. 2010). However, during the late 1990s, public interest in bullying intensified as a series of high-profile school shootings in the United States implicated bullying as an underlying cause (Anderson et al. 2001; Stuart-Cassel et al. 2011). National media outlets now cover incidents of bullying with regularity. Movies, television programs, and social media have helped to raise awareness and provide a voice to bullying victims. Unfortunately, some of the outlets used to combat bullying (e.g., social media) serve as a vector for its perpetration (Luxton et al. 2012). For example, we have all heard about tragedies in which online bullying was a contributing factor to suicide. Television programs that sensationalize suicide in bullied youth coupled with the use of social media as a forum for publicizing self-harm and suicide in response to bullying raise concern for the "contagion effect" that places more youth in harm's way (Zarghami 2012).

Concurrent with the heightened visibility of the issue of bullying, there has been a marked increase in research establishing a link between bullying and long-term health consequences, such as depression, substance use, aggression, and school truancy (Brunstein Klomek et al. 2007; Copeland et al. 2013; Gastic 2008; Juvonen et al. 2011; Nansel et al. 2001; O'Brennan et al. 2009; Roland 2002). Modern-day perspectives of bullying as a serious, detrimental, and urgent issue have largely replaced traditional views that these behaviors are merely part of a "rite of passage."

Definition and Types of Bullying

Bullying is a complex emotional and social phenomenon involving the deliberate infliction of harm wherein the bully leverages an advantage (e.g., in physical strength or popularity) over the victim (Smith et al. 2002). For decades, researchers relied on the work of Dr. Daniel Olweus (1996, 2001) to define *bullying* as 1) aggressive behaviors that 2) are repeated and 3) involve an observed or perceived power imbalance favoring the perpetrator. Accordingly, bullying includes the intentional and repetitive harm or injury of a victim who is unable to defend himself or herself within the context of these power imbalances.

As bullying becomes increasingly salient within legal and public health spheres, its definition continues to evolve. In 2014, the Centers for Disease Control and Prevention and the U.S. Department of Education released the first uniform definition of bullying for public health research and surveillance, highlighting it as a distinct entity from other forms of violence among youth such as dating violence or gang violence (Hunter et al. 2007). The definition is as follows:

TABLE 5–1. Main forms of bullying

Type of bullying	Type of behaviors	Examples
Verbal	Spoken behaviors	Name-calling, taunting, inappropriate comments
Physical	Body gestures	Hitting, kicking, damaging someone's property
Psychological	Relational aggression	Embarrassing someone, excluding others from activities
Cyber	Online bullying	Mean text messages, posting rumors on social media
Sexual	All of the above	Sexual jokes or innuendo, gestures, unwelcome looks or touching

> Bullying is any unwanted aggressive behavior(s) by another youth or group of youths who are not siblings or current dating partners that involves an observed or perceived power imbalance and is repeated multiple times or is highly likely to be repeated. Bullying may inflict harm or distress on the targeted youth including physical, psychological, social, or educational harm. (Gladden et al. 2014, p. 7)

This definition distinguishes bullying from other forms of aggressive behavior that are unlikely to be repeated or that do not involve a power imbalance. This precision of language is important for understanding long-term outcomes. For example, peer victimization (i.e., when a child is the repeated target of aggression by peers) and bullying (i.e., repeated acts of aggression intended to cause harm or psychological distress in the context of a power differential between aggressor and victim) have long been conceptualized as indistinct; it is now known that these concepts are qualitatively different experiences among youth, and bullying leads to more depressive symptomatology compared with peer victimization (Hunter et al. 2007).

The definition of bullying has important legal ramifications, and public attention has been anchored in the tragedies publicized in the media. Stories of extreme bullying, school shootings, and suicides have propelled most states to enact antibullying legislation (Srabstein et al. 2008; Stuart-Cassel et al. 2011). New legal regulations have been used to deter and punish bullying, and research has led to the development of numerous public health models that work to reduce this phenomenon (Ttofi et al. 2011). Bullying exists worldwide and across all age groups and remains one of many problems youths face (Magnuson and Norem 2009).

The main forms of bullying are verbal, physical, psychological, and cyber (see Table 5–1).

Verbal bullying refers to the use of spoken behaviors to inflect harm on an individual. Examples include teasing, name-calling, making inappropriate sexual comments, and taunting.

Physical bullying is the use of gestures or actions to threaten or inflict harm. Hitting, kicking, punching, spitting, pushing, using offensive gestures, and damaging someone else's property are examples of physical bullying.

Psychological bullying is a form of relational aggression that targets the victim's reputation or relationships. Characteristic examples include spreading rumors, purposefully excluding others from activities, withholding friendship, and intentionally embarrassing someone in public (Crick and Grotpeter 1995).

Cyberbullying is a relatively recent phenomenon that has evolved alongside the Net Gen—a term used to describe individuals born after 1982—and the expansion of electronic socialization. It is defined as the use of technology, through social networking sites, e-mails, websites, chats, online forums, or text messages, to support hostile behaviors intended to harm others (Butler et al. 2009). Examples of cyberbullying include antagonistic text messages or e-mails, rumors spread via e-mail or posted on social networking sites, embarrassing pictures or videos, and fake profiles. Although there is a conceptual overlap between cyberbullying and traditional forms of bullying, there are several key differences. The content of cyberbullying can be quickly disseminated and made available to an almost infinite number of people via the Internet. Moreover, cyberbullying does not require physical strength, and perpetrators can rely on such advantages as ability to navigate social media, anonymity, and the victim's limited defenses (Dehue et al. 2008). It extends the reach of school bullying beyond school grounds and into the digital sphere. Social media has become recognized as a vehicle through which youth can perpetuate bullying of peers off school grounds as well as providing an arena to show a suicide, which is termed *cybersuicide* (Biddle et al. 2018; Luxton et al. 2012).

Bullying can be sexual in nature, with *sexual bullying* involving a power dynamic in which the perpetrator intends harm to the victim. Examples of sexual bullying include sexual jokes or comments, gestures, looks, touching, exposing, or rumors. Under the law, sexual bullying is distinct from sexual harassment, which has legal consequences. *Sexual harassment* is a broad term for unwanted behavior that is sexual in nature (Miller and Mondschein 2017; Stein 2003). Schools have a legal responsibility to create a safe learning environment and are liable in cases of harassment. On the other hand, bullying entails liability of the culprit. The distinction between the two behaviors may be important with regard to potential legal implications.

Early research on bullying dichotomized youth into two groups: bully and victim. However, it has become clear that some youth fall into both categories—that is, they are both bullying others and the victims of bullying themselves. This group has been identified as *bully/victim* and has led to the use of a more accurate model of a bully/victim continuum (Bosworth et al. 1999; Haynie et al. 2001; Swearer et al. 2001).

Prevalence

Longitudinal studies demonstrate that bullying starts as early as elementary school but is most prevalent in middle school and early adolescence. Rates of middle school bullying as high as 81% have been reported (Bosworth et al. 1999).

Bullying prevalence estimates vary widely because of differing definitions, strategies for assessment, and sample characteristics; however, rates of bullying are far from insignificant (Brochado et al. 2017). Estimates of the prevalence of school bullying in the United States are derived from national surveys, including the Health Behaviors in School-age Children (HBSC), the School Crime Supplement (SCS) to the National Crime Victimization Survey, and the Youth Risk Behavior Surveillance System (YRBSS). These assessments of bullying suggest that about one in five youth experience bullying at any given time (Brochado et al. 2017; Gladden et al. 2014; Kann et al. 2017). The 2017 YRBSS, based on a sample of youth in grades 9–12, reported that 19% of students had been bullied during the 12 months preceding the survey. Although bullying generally decreases in later adolescence, some youth exhibit more bullying behaviors throughout adolescence (Rettew and Pawlowski 2016).

Most, but not all, studies report that males engage in more frequent bullying compared with females (Bosworth et al. 1999). Males are more likely to engage in physical forms of bullying, whereas females engage in more psychological bullying and relational aggression (Crick and Grotpeter 1995; Wang et al. 2009). With regard to cyberbullying, females are more often the victims, and males are more often the bullies. The sites of bullying and victimization also appear to differ between males and females. The 2015 SCS suggested that males may be bullied more frequently on the school bus, outside (on school grounds), or in a bathroom or locker room, whereas females were more likely to be bullied online or by text (U.S. Department of Education 2016). Among the youth from the 2017 YRBSS sample, 19% of females reported bullying on school property, compared with 15.6% of their male counterparts (Kann et al. 2017).

Bullying and cyberbullying often co-occur, and studies demonstrate that cyberbullying has become a growing problem. Among middle and high school students, as many as 33% report bullying others online, and

50% have been victims of cyberbullying (Hinduja and Patchin 2013; Mishna et al. 2010). According to a review of 36 studies, mostly based in the United States, the median prevalence of cyberbullying was 23% (range 11%–43%) among adolescents between ages 12 and 18 (Hamm et al. 2015).

Contributing Factors

Involvement in bullying, as aggressor or victim, may have some temporal stability, but youth appear to fluctuate between perpetrator and victim roles over time and according to specific circumstances (Gumpel et al. 2014; Ryoo et al. 2015). Studies of elementary school victims of bullying suggest that 15%–43% were still being bullied 4 years later (Kumpulainen et al. 1999; Scholte et al. 2007). The course of bullying behaviors may be explained, in part, by the reciprocal influences between risk factors. For example, internalizing behaviors are a risk factor for bullying, but victims of bullying are also more likely to develop internalizing behaviors. This creates a vicious cycle that contributes to the perpetuation of bullying and victimization. Chronically bullied youth may have distinct risk factors and outcomes and are at greatest risk for developing poor outcomes (Barker et al. 2008).

Individual and contextual factors—namely, home and school environment—confer risk to the development of bullying behaviors, although this risk varies across age, race/ethnicity, and gender groups (Swearer Napolitano 2011; Spriggs et al. 2007). A brief overview of associated factors is found in Table 5–2.

Characteristics of Bullies and Victims

Who are the typical bullies and victims of bullying? Bullies tend to have been exposed to family conflict and generally target peers with actual or perceived differences. Victims may appear overweight or underweight, wear glasses or different clothing, or be unable to afford what others consider "cool." Other differences include being new to a school, being less popular and having few friends, or having a disability. Sexual orientation, race, and gender are also common differences that relate to bullying behaviors. In this section, we review some common characteristics among youth who bully and the victims of bullying. It is important to note that bullying often creates a vicious cycle, with bullying begetting more bullying. It is not unusual for a young person to be both a perpetrator and a victim.

School Settings

Negative school climate (i.e., lower degree of respect and fair treatment of students and lower sense of belonging) is associated with greater risk

TABLE 5–2. **General associations in risk factors for bullying**

Bully	Victim	References
More externalizing behaviors (e.g., aggression, misconduct)	More internalizing behaviors (e.g., depression, anxiety)	Hodges and Perry 1999
More social competence, friendship protection	Poorer relationships	Wang et al. 2009
Domestic violence	Harsh, reactive parenting	Bowes et al. 2009

of bully perpetration and victimization (Cook et al. 2010). Youth who perceive a connection with their schools and a positive school climate report less involvement in bullying (Williams and Guerra 2007). Larger schools may also have greater rates of victimization compared with smaller schools (Bowes et al. 2009). However, children in smaller classes may be victimized more often (Wolke et al. 2001).

On the Home Front

Harsh and reactive parenting styles, characterized by coercive acts and negative emotional expressions toward children (e.g., yelling, spanking, hitting), are associated with high and chronic levels of peer victimization (Arseneault et al. 2010; Barker et al. 2008; Chang et al. 2003; Erath et al. 2009). Positive parental behaviors seem to protect youth from bullying others and being bullied (Espelage et al. 2001; Wang et al. 2009).

Family conflict is also associated with increased rates of bully perpetration and victimization (Cook et al. 2010; Swearer et al. 2001). Domestic violence, in particular, may be a risk factor for becoming a bully (Bowes et al. 2009). Maternal deprivation and lower socioeconomic status may be linked to higher rates of bullying and victimization, although there are conflicting data on this association (Bowers et al. 1994; Tippett and Wolke 2014).

Parental substance use is associated with increased bully perpetration and victimization (Cook et al. 2010; Swearer et al. 2001). Youth whose mothers have a mental health problem are more likely to become victims of bullying compared with their peers (Wolke et al. 2001).

Bullying as a Vicious Cycle

Prior victimization is a risk factor for being bullied and is common among bully perpetrators (Kljakovic and Hunt 2016; Wolke et al. 2001). In regard to online bullying, a meta-analysis of 81 empirical studies of cyberbullying showed that traditional bullying perpetration and victimization predict cyberbullying perpetration and victimization, respectively (Chen et al. 2017). Thus, more traditional forms of bullying commonly go hand in hand with cyberbullying.

Sexual Orientation

Youth identifying as lesbian, gay, bisexual, or transgender (LGBT) report higher levels of victimization, including physical violence and injury, compared with non-LGBT peers (Berlan et al. 2010; Bontempo and D'Augelli 2002; Garofalo et al. 1998). In a 2009 study of 7,621 students between ages 13 and 21, LGBT students reported verbal harassment at a rate of 84.6%, physical harassment at a rate of 40.1%, and physical assault at a rate of 18.8% in the prior year (Kosciw et al. 2010).

Internalizing and Externalizing Behaviors

Children with internalizing behaviors, such as anxiety and withdrawal, may be more likely to become victims of bullying (Arseneault et al. 2006; Bollmer et al. 2005; Hodges and Perry 1999). This may be explained by the notion that anxious children can be easy targets and lack the interpersonal effectiveness to navigate peer conflict (Arseneault et al. 2010). On the other hand, there is literature to suggest that bullies and bully/victims are more likely than victims to be depressed (Swearer et al. 2001). Cyberbully perpetrators, in particular, have higher rates of depression compared with cyberbully victims (Chen et al. 2017). Externalizing symptoms, such as delinquency and aggression, are more common in bully perpetrators (Cook et al. 2010; Ivarsson et al. 2005).

Anger, Aggression, and Impulsivity

Children's emotional orientation is also an important risk factor for the development of bullying behavior. Youth with high levels of anger, impulsivity, and hyperactivity are more likely to bully others (Bosworth et al. 1999; Espelage et al. 2001; Farrington and Baldry 2010). Early childhood aggressiveness is associated with peer rejection and increased risk of victimization, which can lead to psychological distress and hostility (Barker et al. 2008; Ladd and Troop-Gordon 2003). Bullying may stem from attempts to cope with strong emotions such as anger and depression. Youth from chaotic homes may use bullying to feel a sense of control in what otherwise feels unpredictable and unsafe. Moral acceptability of bullying is associated with greater rates of bullying perpetration (Williams and Guerra 2007). Youth with beliefs supportive of violence and misconduct are more likely to become bullies (Bosworth et al. 1999; Chen et al. 2017; Espelage et al. 2001).

TABLE 5–3. **Key outcomes of bullying and victimization**

	Bullies	Victims	References
Psychological outcomes	Depression Suicidal ideation	Depression Suicidal ideation Anxiety Poor perceived quality of life	Arseneault et al. 2006; Takizawa et al. 2014
Biological outcomes	Substance use	Substance use Poorer health outcomes	Kaltiala-Heino et al. 2000; Moore et al. 2017; Nansel et al. 2001; Takizawa et al. 2014
Social outcomes	Street crime Violent injury Dating violence	More likely to become bully/ victims Lower educational attainment	Andershed et al. 2001; Connolly et al. 2000; Haynie et al. 2001

Peer Status

The function of social status may be explained by the *friendship protection hypothesis*, which suggests that having friends protects an individual from becoming the target of bullying (Boulton et al. 1999; Hodges and Perry 1999; Spriggs et al. 2007). When youth perceive peers as trustworthy, caring, and helpful, they report less engagement in bullying, which supports the notion of bullying as a reaction to perceived danger and hostility (Williams and Guerra 2007). Youth with poorer relationships are at increased risk of becoming victims or bully/victims (Cook et al. 2010). Youth with more friends may be less vulnerable to aggressive peers and may be more likely to become bullies. Bullies tend to be less socially isolated and gain popularity more easily, especially among other aggressive peers (Wang et al. 2009).

Outcomes of Bullying and Victimization

Youth involved in bullying as bullies, victims, and bystanders endure negative effects that carry into adulthood (Eron et al. 1987). Cross-sectional studies of elementary school, middle school, and high school students show that bullies, victims, and bully/victims experience greater psychological distress than their counterparts do (Arseneault et al. 2006; Kim et al. 2005; van der Wal et al. 2003). The consequences of bullying involvement commonly persist into adulthood (Takizawa et al. 2014). The key findings are outlined in Table 5–3.

Bullies, victims, and bully/victims report higher rates of depression, suicidal ideation, and suicidal behaviors compared with peers not involved in bullying (Arseneault et al. 2010; Bauman et al. 2013; Brunstein Klomek et al. 2007; Kaltiala-Heino et al. 2000; Kim et al. 2009; Klomek et al. 2008, 2009; Nansel et al. 2001; Roland 2002; Wang et al. 2009; Wolke et al. 2001). Longitudinal data corroborate these findings and show that the experience of being frequently bullied in childhood is associated with increased risk of depression and anxiety disorders as well as suicidality during middle adulthood (Takizawa et al. 2014). There may also be an association between history of traumatic experience of bullying victimization and the development of psychotic symptoms among certain individuals (Bebbington et al. 2004; Janssen et al. 2004; Lataster et al. 2006). Bullies and victims are more likely to engage in alcohol, tobacco, and illicit drug use (Kaltiala-Heino et al. 2000; Moore et al. 2017; Nansel et al. 2001; Pepler et al. 2002). Victims of bullying have lower grade point averages, higher dropout rates, and more frequent absences from school compared with their peers (Gastic 2008; Juvonen et al. 2011; Schwartz and Hopmeyer Gorman 2003). A study of bully victims followed into adulthood showed that those who experienced bullying victimization as children were at lower educational levels at midlife (Takizawa et al. 2014). Victims of bullying have poorer health outcomes and lower perceived quality of life as adults (Moore et al. 2017; Rigby 1999). History of bullying is a risk factor associated with sustaining violent injuries, engaging in dating violence, and participating in street crime (Andershed et al. 2001; Connolly et al. 2000). Interestingly, chronic victims of bullying have a higher risk of becoming bullies themselves (Haynie et al. 2001; Smokowski and Kopasz 2005). Childhood bully/victims may be more likely to engage in criminal offenses during late adolescence, but the potential for violence may differ on the basis of type of bullying behavior. For example, a study by Lindberg et al. (2012) found that adolescents who make threats online were at greater risk for intending to commit the violent act when compared with adolescents who make threats off-line (Lindberg et al. 2012).

Strategies to Address Bullying and Cyberbullying at School

When developing policies to curtail bullying, schools must consider state, federal, and local regulations as well as potential challenges related to civil rights laws, protections of free speech, and new trends such as cyberbullying (Ttofi et al. 2011). Laws on bullying and cyberbullying vary around the country, which contributes to complexities in creating school policies. Many state laws include the condition that the bullying creates a hostile educational environment or refer to the "reasonable person" as a comparative standard for determining whether a behavior constitutes bullying (Stuart-Cassel et al. 2011). In the following subsection, we discuss two of several landmark legal cases that provide context for the evolution of antibullying policies in schools.

Case Law

Tinker v. Des Moines Independent Community School District (1969)

In 1965, five youth from Des Moines, Iowa planned to wear black armbands to school to protest the United States' involvement in the Vietnam War. Word of the students' plan spread to the children's respective school principals, who immediately instituted a district-wide policy that forbade students from wearing armbands as a form of political protest. All five children, who ranged in age from 8 to 16 years, chose to violate this new policy, and the three oldest participants were suspended. The Iowa Civil Liberties Union became involved, and a lawsuit was filed. The school board's decision was upheld in both U.S. District Court and the 8th Circuit Court of Appeals. The U.S. Supreme Court ultimately ruled that the students' suspension for wearing black armbands in protest of the Vietnam War violated their First Amendment right to free speech. The disruptive behavior that occurred on campus was deemed passive and nonthreatening. The *Tinker* case set a precedent that the First Amendment protects the right of students to express controversial views that diverge from official school policy, as long as they do not cause "material and substantial interference with schoolwork or discipline" or represent an "invasion of the rights of others" (Tinker v. Des Moines Independent Community School District 1969).

Since the Tinker decision, the right to free speech has been a relevant consideration in later cases as a factor to defend bullying behavior (e.g., J.S. v. Bethlehem Area School District 2002; Morse v. Frederick 2007). Courts are asked to decide whether student behavior is protected as free speech, and outcomes have varied. Further examples of cases related to bullying are provided in the following subsections.

Kowalski v. Berkeley County School District (2011)

In the case of Kowalski v. Berkeley County School District (2011), a high school student from West Virginia, Ms. Kowalski, was suspended from school for creating a web page titled "S.A.S.H." or "Students Against Sluts Herpes" that was used as a forum for slandering a fellow student. The female victim and her parents filed a complaint with the school's administration, who characterized Ms. Kowalski's web page as a "hate website." Ms. Kowalski received a 5-day suspension from class and a 90-day suspension from extracurricular activities. Ms. Kowalski filed a lawsuit claiming that the school's disciplinary actions violated her First Amendment rights to free speech and due process. The district court upheld the school's decision to suspend Ms. Kowalski, and the appeals court ultimately concluded that the school had the right to discipline students whose actions interfered with the operation of the school and infringed on the rights of fellow students.

People v. Marquan (2014)

In 2010, a high school student from Cohoes, New York posted pictures of classmates and associated lewd comments on Facebook. A month prior, the Albany County Legislature outlawed cyberbullying by making "any act of communicating...with the intent to harass, annoy, threaten, abuse, taunt, intimidate, torment, humiliate, or otherwise inflict significant emotional harm on another person" a misdemeanor offense punishable by up to a year in jail and a $1000 fine (People v. Marquan 2014). The student was charged under the new law, and his attempts to have the case dismissed were unsuccessful. The student eventually pleaded guilty, then filed an appeal arguing that the law violated protections for free speech afforded by the First Amendment. The New York Court of Appeals agreed with the student, ruling that "the text of Albany County's law envelops far more than acts of cyberbullying against children by criminalizing a variety of constitutionally-protected modes of expression" (People v. Marquan 2014).

State v. Bishop (2016)

North Carolina passed legislation in 2009 that made cyberbullying of minors a criminal offense. In 2011, a high school student from Alamance County, North Carolina posted several derogatory comments about a classmate on Facebook. The classmate's mother discovered the offensive comments, then notified local law enforcement officials, who gathered screenshots of the comments using an undercover Facebook account. A jury found the student who posted the negative comments guilty of one count of cyberbullying. He received a suspended sentence of 30 days in the custody of the Alamance County Sheriff and was placed on 48 months of supervised probation. The defendant appealed his conviction, and the case made its way to the Supreme Court of North Carolina, which ruled that "the statute violates the First Amendment as applied to the states through the Fourteenth Amendment" and "sweeps far beyond the State's legitimate interest in protecting the psychological health of minors" (State v. Bishop 2016).

Davis v. Monroe County Board of Education (1999)

Despite recent case law suggesting that cyberbullying is protected speech under the First Amendment, this is a complex issue that is far from resolved. In the case of Davis v. Monroe County Board of Education (1999), a fifth-grade girl from Georgia was repeatedly sexually harassed by a classmate despite telling school officials what was happening to her. The child's mother sued the school board, and the case was eventually heard by the U.S. Supreme Court. Justice Sandra Day O'Connor's majority opinion held that schools are liable for monetary damages when staff behave in a manner that is "deliberately indifferent to sexual harassment, of which they have actual knowledge, that harassment is so severe, pervasive, and objectively offensive that it can be said to deprive the victims of access to the educational opportunities or benefits provided by the school." The term *deliberate indifference* applies when school officials are aware of harassment yet choose to ignore it and/or repeatedly address it in a manner that has been clearly demonstrated to be ineffective.

Does the Davis case, along with the language in Tinker protecting speech as long as it does not interfere with schoolwork or invade the rights of others, set the stage for school districts that ignore cyberbullying to be held liable for monetary damages? This scenario places schools between a rock and a hard place given that disciplining students who engage in off-campus cyberbullying may result in claims that the cyberbullies' actions are protected speech under the First Amendment. In our opinion, schools must be able to intervene in cases of cyberbullying that clearly interfere with students' well-being; however, making such determinations in a transparent and bias-free manner may be easier said than done.

School-Based Intervention

In addition to the legal implications of creating school-based bullying interventions, effectiveness is another key consideration. Some programs have demonstrated effectiveness in reducing the incidence of bullying (Black and Jackson 2007; Kellam et al. 2011; Salmivalli et al. 2011), and interventions have varying success rates depending on the methodology and population studied (Bauer et al. 2007; Merrell et al. 2008; Olweus 1996; Ttofi et al. 2011). A systematic review of 44 program evaluations comparing the results of antibullying programs with control groups showed that school-based bullying programs may indeed decrease bullying behaviors (Ttofi et al. 2011). Program intensity and duration, parent involvement, and playground supervision were among some of the factors associated with increased program effectiveness. The most effective programs address larger social factors and do not focus exclusively on the individuals engaging in or experiencing the bullying behaviors (Bradshaw et al. 2007; Espelage and Swearer 2010; Hamburger et al. 2011; Swearer and Doll 2001).

Other research suggests that prevention programs can have positive influences on knowledge and attitudes about bullying but may not actually reduce bullying behaviors (Merrell et al. 2008). In a meta-analysis of 16 studies of bullying intervention across the United States and Europe,

Merrell and colleagues found that bullying interventions were associated with meaningful changes in several outcomes, including improved social competence, self-esteem, and peer acceptance, but did not demonstrate meaningful impact on the occurrence of bullying. Thus, interpretation of the data from bullying interventions must be considered in the context of certain limitations, including variability in methodology of interventions, heterogeneity of student bodies and family influences, diversity of school characteristics, and general difficulty implementing school-wide programs. Nonetheless, bullying behaviors tend to increase without appropriate intervention (Olweus 1994).

Given the association between bullying behaviors and suicide risk and research demonstrating the effectiveness of school-based suicide prevention programs, comprehensive prevention efforts have been the subject of public health discussion (Centers for Disease Control and Prevention, National Center for Injury Prevention and Control 2008; Merrell et al. 2008; Zenere and Lazarus 1997). Primary strategies to prevent suicide and bullying include the identification of at-risk youth, promotion of social support, and reduction of social isolation.

Approaches to school-based bullying prevention vary widely from purely curricular programs to more comprehensive programs geared toward changing the school climate. Nationally recognized tools have been developed to assist in evaluating the effectiveness of these school-based interventions (Thornton et al. 2002). Much of what we have learned about bullying intervention is informed by the shortcomings of prior interventions, such as zero-tolerance or three-strikes-and-you're-out policies that suspend or expel bullies. We now know that these policies typically are ineffective at deterring repeat aggression, and the threat of suspension or expulsion may inadvertently discourage youth from reporting bullying (Ayers et al. 2012). Other interventions such as conflict resolution and peer mediation may inadvertently send the message that both parties are at fault rather than teaching that the bullying behavior is inappropriate (Limber 2003). Another important consideration is that excessive focus on issues of mental health and suicide may contribute to contagion processes whereby youth start to engage in the behaviors being discussed in light of the perception that they may garner power and/or attention. Episodic prevention efforts, such as school-wide assemblies, brief campaigns, or parent-teacher association meetings, are unlikely to foster lasting changes in bullying behaviors (StopBullying.gov 2017). It is also important to note that prevention programs that target physical fighting and aggression are unsuccessful in preventing bullying behaviors (Van Schoiack-Edstrom et al. 2002).

The most effective bullying interventions involve widespread changes in the school climate, with highly involved teachers and parents and consistent disciplining of bullying behaviors (Eliot et al. 2010;

TABLE 5–4. **Key elements of effective versus ineffective school-based bullying interventions**

Effective interventions	Ineffective interventions
High levels of playground supervision	Zero-tolerance policies
Rules related to bullying	Grouping bullies together (e.g., in
Trained teachers	group therapy)
Involved parents	Brief awareness campaigns

Gottfredson and DiPietro 2011; Gottfredson et al. 2005; Gregory et al. 2010). Interventions should aim to make victims of bullying feel safe at school (Seeley et al. 2011). Despite the experience of being bullied, victims of bullying must hold hope for the future with the sense that they can overcome the challenge. Bullies and victims should be surrounded by responsible adults who can model caring and appropriate behaviors, especially because youths' access to adult role models outside school may be limited. The key elements of effective and ineffective interventions are outlined in Table 5–4.

One of the most widely implemented and best researched models for bullying prevention is the Olweus Bullying Prevention Program (OBPP; Olweus 1996; Olweus and Limber 2010). OBPP is an internationally recognized school-based program that involves individual, classroom, school-wide, and community components. The long-term goal is to create a safe, positive school climate by reducing and preventing bullying as well as improving peer relations. This is accomplished by setting firm limits to unacceptable behaviors and consistently applying nonhostile, noncorporeal sanctions when rules are violated. The program is unique in that it involves all adults within the school environment (i.e., teachers, parents, administrators, nonteaching staff). The impetus for change is through actively involved adults who act simultaneously as authority figures and positive role models, conveying the message "Bullying is not accepted in our class and school, and we will see to it that it comes to an end." OBPP is designed for use with students in grades 3 through 10. A number of studies have demonstrated the program's effectiveness in reducing the incidence of bullying, with some reductions as high as 65% over the course of 4 years (Black and Jackson 2007; Olweus et al. 1999). See Table 5–5 for a program overview.

Bully Busters is another evidence-based school-wide bullying intervention (Newman-Carlson et al. 2000). The program is based on the premise that bullying arises from deficits in a child's social skills. It focuses on empowering teachers to effectively detect, prevent, and manage bullying behaviors. There are separate manuals for elementary, middle, and high school teachers and staff as well as a parent guide. Several studies

TABLE 5–5. Olweus Bullying Prevention Program

School	Classroom	Student
Bullying prevention committee meets regularly to supervise the project and secure community involvement	Engage students in activities such as role-playing to illustrate harms related to bullying	Support victims
Administer a school-wide survey to determine the current status of bullying, including times and kinds of bullying occurrences	Encourage students to explore ways to decrease bullying	Provide interventions for bullies
Increase teacher supervision during likely times and locations of bullying	Intervene when bullying behavior is detected	Meet with student and parents if bullying behavior occurs

Source.   Olweus 1996; https://olweus.sites.clemson.edu.

support the use of Bully Busters and demonstrate a reduction in classroom bullying and improvement in teacher self-efficacy related to intervention skills (Newman-Carlson and Horne 2004; Orpinas et al. 2003).

For a noncomprehensive list of research-informed bullying interventions, see Table 5–6. Additional resources on bullying can be found at www.stopbullying.gov/prevention/at-school/index.html.

Importantly, some literature shows that school-based prevention programs are less effective in the United States than in other countries (Farrington and Ttofi 2009). Thus, it is critical that bullying interventions are not limited to the school setting and that institutions carefully consider which interventions are most appropriate given the student body, school, and community characteristics. Nationally based registries of evidence-based interventions are valuable resources in selecting an appropriate bullying intervention. The following are recommended:

- Blueprints for Healthy Youth Development (www.colorado.edu/cspv/blueprints)
- Evidence-Based Practices Resource Center (www.samhsa.gov/ebp-resource-center)
- Model Programs Guide (www.ojjdp.gov/mpg)

TABLE 5–6.   Research-informed bullying interventions

Program	Overview and method	Website
Al's Pals: Kids Making Healthy Choices (Lynch et al. 2003)	Develops problem solving, healthy decision making, and self-control	http://wingspanworks.com/healthy-al
Allan L. Beane Bullying Prevention Program (Beane 2009; Spurling 2004)	Promotes acceptance of and belonging for all individuals	www.bullyfree.com/school-program/description-of-the-bullying-prevention-program
Bully Busters (Newman-Carlson et al. 2000)	Improves teacher awareness and intervention skills	www.researchpress.com/books/455/bully-busters
Good Behavior Game (Kellam et al. 2011)	Provides classroom management strategies to reward children for demonstrating on-task behaviors	www.goodbehaviorgame.org
KiVa (Salmivalli et al. 2011)	Engages bystanders by increasing antibullying attitudes	www.kivaprogram.net
Life Skills Training (Botvin et al. 2006)	Targets psychological and social factors that promote problematic behaviors	https://lifeskillstraining.com
Olweus Bullying Prevention Program (Olweus and Limber 2010)	Encourages school-wide awareness of bullying to improve peer relations and promote positive school environment	https://olweus.sites.clemson.edu
Open Circle (Hennessey 2007; Taylor et al. 2002)	Fosters social-emotional learning and positive relationships	www.open-circle.org
PeaceBuilders (Flannery et al. 2003; Vazsonyi et al. n.d.)	Encourages transformation of school climate through setting behavioral expectations and modeling a positive culture	www.peacebuilders.com
Safe School Ambassadors (White et al. 2011)	Trains bystanders to serve as ambassadors and positively shape social climate	https://community-matters.org/programs-and-services/safe-school-ambassadors
Second Step Bullying Prevention Unit (Committee for Children 2013)	Teaches youth social-emotional skills for bullying prevention	www.secondstep.org/bullying-prevention#research-materials-section

Conclusion

In summary, bullying and cyberbullying are known to have serious and long-lasting negative effects. Our review of legal cases from around the country shows that, in general, schools are on solid ground when they take actions that are deemed to be in the best interest of bullying victims and to protect the student body at large.

National attention to bullying, some of which involves the misuse of social media and other digital outlets, is often centered on blame and legal intervention instead of evidence-based action to prevent future behaviors. The increasing body of evidence for the prevalence and impact of bullying underscores the need for prompt corrective action. The present and future welfare of youth depends on prioritizing socially responsible behavior and collaboration between stakeholders (e.g., students, parents, school districts, the media, social media companies).

Key Points

- Concurrent with the heightened visibility of the issue of bullying, there has been a marked increase in research establishing the link between bullying and long-term health consequences, such as depression, substance use, aggression, and school truancy.

- The function of social status may be explained by the friendship protection hypothesis, which suggests that having friends protects an individual from becoming the target of bullying.

- Cyberbullying extends the reach of school bullying beyond school grounds and into the digital sphere.

- The most effective bullying interventions involve widespread changes in the school climate, with highly involved teachers and parents and consistent discipline of bullying behaviors.

Clinical Pearls

Understanding the definition of bullying is important for differentiating it from other forms of aggression and to understand outcomes associated with bullying. The Centers for Disease Control and Prevention and U.S. Department of Education have a unified definition for bullying. *Bullying* is any unwanted aggressive behavior(s) by another youth or group of youths who are not siblings or current dating partners that involves an observed or perceived power imbalance and is repeated multiple times or is highly likely to be repeated. Bullying may inflict harm or distress on the targeted youth, including physical, psychological, social, or educational harm.

Involvement in bullying, as aggressor or victim, may have some temporal stability, but youth appear to fluctuate between perpetrator and victim roles over time and according to specific circumstances.

Bullies and victims should be surrounded by responsible adults who can model caring and appropriate behaviors, especially because youth access to adult role models outside school may be limited.

References

Andershed H, Kerr M, Stattin H: Bullying in school and violence on the streets: are the same people involved? J Scand Stud Criminol Crime Prev 2(1):31–49, 2001

Anderson M, Kaufman J, Simon TR, et al: School-associated violent deaths in the United States, 1994–1999. JAMA 286(21):2695–2702, 2001 11730445

Arseneault L, Bowes L, Shakoor S: Bullying victimization in youths and mental health problems: 'much ado about nothing'? Psychol Med 40(5):717–729, 2010 19785920

Arseneault L, Walsh E, Trzesniewski K, et al: Bullying victimization uniquely contributes to adjustment problems in young children: a nationally representative cohort study. Pediatrics 118(1):130–138, 2006 16818558

Ayers SL, Wagaman MA, Geiger JM, et al: Examining school-based bullying interventions using multilevel discrete time hazard modeling. Prev Sci 13(5):539–550, 2012 22878779

Barker ED, Boivin M, Brendgen M, et al: Predictive validity and early predictors of peer-victimization trajectories in preschool. Arch Gen Psychiatry 65(10):1185–1192, 2008 18838635

Bauer NS, Lozano P, Rivara FP: The effectiveness of the Olweus Bullying Prevention Program in public middle schools: a controlled trial. J Adolesc Health 40(3):266–274, 2007 17321428

Bauman S, Toomey RB, Walker JL: Associations among bullying, cyberbullying, and suicide in high school students. J Adolesc 36(2):341–350, 2013 23332116

Beane AL: Bullying Prevention for Schools: A Step-by-Step Guide to Implementing a Successful Anti-Bullying Program. San Francisco, CA, Jossey-Bass, 2009

Bebbington PE, Bhugra D, Brugha T, et al: Psychosis, victimisation and childhood disadvantage: evidence from the second British National Survey of Psychiatric Morbidity. Br J Psychiatry 185(03):220–226, 2004 15339826

Berlan ED, Corliss HL, Field AE, et al: Sexual orientation and bullying among adolescents in the Growing Up Today Study. J Adolesc Health 46(4):366–371, 2010 20307826

Biddle L, Derges J, Goldsmith C, et al: Using the Internet for suicide-related purposes: contrasting findings from young people in the community and self-harm patients admitted to hospital. PLoS One 13(5):e0197712, 2018 29795637

Black SA, Jackson E: Using bullying incident density to evaluate the Olweus Bullying Prevention Programme. Sch Psychol Int 28(5):623–638, 2007

Bollmer JM, Milich R, Harris MJ, Maras MA: A friend in need: the role of friendship quality as a protective factor in peer victimization and bullying. J Interpers Violence 20(6):701–712, 2005 15851537

Bontempo DE, D'Augelli AR: Effects of at-school victimization and sexual orientation on lesbian, gay, or bisexual youths' health risk behavior. J Adolesc Health 30(5):364–374, 2002 11996785

Bosworth K, Espelage DL, Simon TR: Factors associated with bullying behavior in middle school students. J Early Adolesc 19(3):341–362, 1999

Botvin GJ, Griffin KW, Diaz Nichols Botvin T: Preventing youth violence and delinquency through a universal school-based prevention approach. Prev Sci 7(4):403–408, 2006 17136462

Boulton MJ, Trueman M, Chau C, et al: Concurrent and longitudinal links between friendship and peer victimization: implications for befriending interventions. J Adolesc 22(4):461–466, 1999 10469510

Bowers L, Smith PK, Binney V: Perceived family relationships of bullies, victims and bully/victims in middle childhood. J Soc Pers Relat 11(2):215–232, 1994

Bowes L, Arseneault L, Maughan B, et al: School, neighborhood, and family factors are associated with children's bullying involvement: a nationally representative longitudinal study. J Am Acad Child Adolesc Psychiatry 48(5):545–553, 2009 19325496

Bradshaw CP, Sawyer AL, O'Brennan LM: Bullying and peer victimization at school: perceptual differences between students and school staff. School Psych Rev 36(3):361–382, 2007

Brochado S, Soares S, Fraga S: A scoping review on studies of cyberbullying prevalence among adolescents. Trauma Violence Abuse 18(5):523–531, 2017 27053102

Brunstein Klomek A, Marrocco F, Kleinman M, et al: Bullying, depression, and suicidality in adolescents. J Am Acad Child Adolesc Psychiatry 46(1):40–49, 2007 17195728

Butler DA, Kift SM, Campbell M, et al: Cyber bullying in schools and the law: is there an effective means of addressing the power imbalance? eLaw Journal 16(1):84–114, 2009

Centers for Disease Control and Prevention, National Center for Injury Prevention and Control: Promoting Individual, Family, and Community Connectedness to Prevent Suicidal: Behavior Strategic Direction for the Prevention of Suicidal Behavior. Atlanta, GA, National Center for Injury Prevention and Control, Centers for Disease Control and Prevention, 2008. Available at: www.cdc.gov/ViolencePrevention/pdf/Suicide_Strategic_Direction_Full_Version-a.pdf. Accessed March 20, 2019.

Chang L, Schwartz D, Dodge KA, et al: Harsh parenting in relation to child emotion regulation and aggression. J Fam Psychol 17(4):598–606, 2003 14640808

Chen L, Ho SS, Lwin MO: A meta-analysis of factors predicting cyberbullying perpetration and victimization: from the social cognitive and media effects approach. New Media Soc 19(8):1194–1213, 2017

Committee for Children: Bullying Prevention Unit: Review of Research. Seattle, WA, Committee for Children, 2013. Available at: www.secondstep.org/Portals/0/common-doc/Review_of_Research_BPU.pdf. Accessed March 20, 2019.

Connolly J, Pepler D, Craig W, et al: Dating experiences of bullies in early adolescence. Child Maltreat 5(4):299–310, 2000 11232258

Cook CR, Williams KR, Guerra NG, et al: Predictors of bullying and victimization in childhood and adolescence: a meta-analytic investigation. School Psychology Quarterly 25(2):65–83, 2010

Copeland WE, Wolke D, Angold A, et al: Adult psychiatric outcomes of bullying and being bullied by peers in childhood and adolescence. JAMA Psychiatry 70(4):419–426, 2013 23426798

Crick NR, Grotpeter JK: Relational aggression, gender, and social-psychological adjustment. Child Dev 66(3):710–722, 1995 7789197

Davis v. Monroe County Board of Education, 526 U.S. 629, 119 S. Ct. 1661, 143 L. Ed. 2d 839 (1999)

Dehue F, Bolman C, Völlink T: Cyberbullying: youngsters' experiences and parental perception. Cyberpsychol Behav 11(2):217–223, 2008 18422417

Eliot M, Cornell D, Gregory A, et al: Supportive school climate and student willingness to seek help for bullying and threats of violence. J Sch Psychol 48(6):533–553, 2010 21094397

Erath SA, El-Sheikh M, Mark Cummings E: Harsh parenting and child externalizing behavior: skin conductance level reactivity as a moderator. Child Dev 80(2):578–592, 2009 19467012

Eron LD, Huesmann LR, Dubow E, et al: Aggression and its correlates over 22 years, in Childhood Aggression and Violence. Edited by Crowell DH, Evans IM, O'Donnell CR. Basingstoke, UK, Springer Nature, 1987, pp 249–262

Espelage DL, Bosworth K, Simon TR: Short-term stability and prospective correlates of bullying in middle-school students: an examination of potential demographic, psychosocial, and environmental influences. Violence Vict 16(4):411–426, 2001 11506450

Espelage DL, Swearer SM: A social-ecological model for bullying prevention and intervention: Understanding the impact of adults in the social ecology of youngsters, in Handbook of Bullying in Schools: An International Perspective. Edited by Jimerson SR, Swearer SM, Espelage DL. New York, Routledge, 2010, pp 61–71

Farrington D, Baldry A: Individual risk factors for school bullying. Journal of Aggression, Conflict, and Peace Research 2(1):4–16, 2010

Farrington DP, Ttofi MM: Reducing school bullying: evidence-based implications for policy. Crime Justice 38(1):281–345, 2009

Flannery DJ, Vazsonyi AT, Liau AK, et al: Initial behavior outcomes for the peacebuilders universal school-based violence prevention program. Dev Psychol 39(2):292–308, 2003 12661887

Garofalo R, Wolf RC, Kessel S, et al: The association between health risk behaviors and sexual orientation among a school-based sample of adolescents. Pediatrics 101(5):895–902, 1998

Gastic B: School truancy and the disciplinary problems of bullying victims. Educational Review 60(4):391–404, 2008

Gladden RM, Vivolo-Kantor AM, Hamburger ME, et al: Bullying Surveillance Among Youths: Uniform Definitions for Public Health and Recommended Data Elements, Version 1.0. Atlanta, GA, National Center for Injury Prevention and Control, Centers for Disease Control and Prevention and U.S. Department of Education, 2014. Available at: https://doi.org/http://www.cdc.gov/violenceprevention/pdf/bullying-definitions-final-a.pdf. Accessed March 20. 2019.

Gottfredson DC, DiPietro SM: School size, social capital, and student victimization. Sociol Educ 84(1):69–89, 2011

Gottfredson GD, Gottfredson DC, Payne AA, et al: School climate predictors of school disorder: results from a national study of delinquency prevention in schools. J Res Crime Delinq 42(4):412–444, 2005

Gregory A, Cornell D, Fan X, et al: Authoritative school discipline: high school practices associated with lower bullying and victimization. J Educ Psychol 102(2):483–496, 2010

Gumpel TP, Zioni-Koren V, Bekerman Z: An ethnographic study of participant roles in school bullying. Aggress Behav 40(3):214–228, 2014 24452451

Hamburger ME, Basile K, Vivolo A: Measuring Bullying Victimization, Perpetration, and Bystander Experiences: A Compendium of Assessment Tools. Atlanta, GA, National Center for Injury Prevention and Control, Centers for Disease Control and Prevention, 2011. Available at: www.cdc.gov/violenceprevention/pdf/bullycompendium-a.pdf. Accessed March 20, 2019.

Hamm MP, Newton AS, Chisholm A, et al: Prevalence and effect of cyberbullying on children and young people: a scoping peview of social media studies. JAMA Pediatr 169(8):770–777, 2015 26098362

Haynie DL, Nansel T, Eitel P, et al: Bullies, victims, and bully/victims. J Early Adolesc 21(1):29–49, 2001

Hennessey BA: Promoting social competence in school-aged children: the effects of the open circle program. J Sch Psychol 45(3):349–360, 2007

Hinduja S, Patchin JW: Social influences on cyberbullying behaviors among middle and high school students. J Youth Adolesc 42(5):711–722, 2013 23296318

Hodges EV, Perry DG: Personal and interpersonal antecedents and consequences of victimization by peers. J Pers Soc Psychol 76(4):677–685, 1999 10234851

Hunter SC, Boyle JME, Warden D: Perceptions and correlates of peer-victimization and bullying. Br J Educ Psychol 77(Pt 4):797–810, 2007 17971286

Ivarsson T, Broberg AG, Arvidsson T, et al: Bullying in adolescence: psychiatric problems in victims and bullies as measured by the Youth Self Report (YSR) and the Depression Self-Rating Scale (DSRS). Nord J Psychiatry 59(5):365–373, 2005 16757465

Janssen I, Krabbendam L, Bak M, et al: Childhood abuse as a risk factor for psychotic experiences. Acta Psychiatr Scand 109(1):38–45, 2004 14674957

J.S. v. Bethlehem Area School District, 807 A.2d 847, 569 Pa. 638 (2002)

Juvonen J, Yueyan Wang Y, Espinoza G: Bullying experiences and compromised academic performance across middle school grades. J Early Adolesc 31(1):152–173, 2011

Kaltiala-Heino R, Rimpelä M, Rantanen P, et al: Bullying at school—an indicator of adolescents at risk for mental disorders. J Adolesc 23(6):661–674, 2000 11161331

Kann L, McManus T, Harris WA, et al: Youth Risk Behavior Surveillance—United States, 2017. MMWR Surveill Summ 67(8):1–114, 2017 29902162

Kellam SG, Mackenzie ACL, Brown CH, et al: The good behavior game and the future of prevention and treatment. Addict Sci Clin Pract 6(1):73–84, 2011 22003425

Kim YS, Koh YJ, Leventhal B: School bullying and suicidal risk in Korean middle school students. Pediatrics 115(2):357–363, 2005 15687445

Kim YS, Leventhal BL, Koh Y-J, Boyce WT: Bullying increased suicide risk: prospective study of Korean adolescents. Arch Suicide Res 13(1):15–30, 2009 19123106

Kljakovic M, Hunt C: A meta-analysis of predictors of bullying and victimisation in adolescence. J Adolesc 49:134–145, 2016 27060847

Klomek AB, Sourander A, Kumpulainen K, et al: Childhood bullying as a risk for later depression and suicidal ideation among Finnish males. J Affect Disord 109(1–2):47–55, 2008 18221788

Klomek AB, Sourander A, Niemelä S, et al: Childhood bullying behaviors as a risk for suicide attempts and completed suicides: a population-based birth cohort study. J Am Acad Child Adolesc Psychiatry 48(3):254–261, 2009 19169159

Kosciw JG, Greytak EA, Diaz EM, et al: The 2009 National School Climate Survey: The Experiences of Lesbian, Gay, Bisexual and Transgender Youth in Our Nation's Schools. New York, GLSEN, 2010. Available at: www.glsen.org/sites/default/files/2009%20National%20School%20Climate%20Survey%20Full%20Report.pdf. Accessed March 20, 2019.

Kowalski v. Berkeley County School District 652 F.3d 565 (4th Cir. 2011)

Kumpulainen K, Räsänen E, Henttonen I: Children involved in bullying: psychological disturbance and the persistence of the involvement. Child Abuse Negl 23(12):1253–1262, 1999 10626609

Ladd GW, Troop-Gordon W: The role of chronic peer difficulties in the development of children's psychological adjustment problems. Child Dev 74(5):1344–1367, 2003 14552402

Lataster T, van Os J, Drukker M, et al: Childhood victimisation and developmental expression of non-clinical delusional ideation and hallucinatory experiences: victimisation and non-clinical psychotic experiences. Soc Psychiatry Psychiatr Epidemiol 41(6):423–428, 2006 16572272

Limber SP: Efforts to address bullying in U.S. schools. Am J Health Educ 34(suppl 5):S23–S29, 2003

Lindberg N, Oksanen A, Sailas E, et al: Adolescents expressing school massacre threats online: something to be extremely worried about? Child Adolesc Psychiatry Ment Health 6(1):39, 2012 23241433

Luxton DD, June JD, Fairall JM: Social media and suicide: a public health perspective. Am J Public Health 102(suppl 2):S195–S200, 2012 22401525

Lynch KB, Geller SR, Schmidt MG: Multi-year evaluation of the effectiveness of a resilience-based prevention program for young children. J Prim Prev 24(3):335–353, 2003

Magnuson S, Norem K: Bullies grow up and go to work. Journal of Professional Counseling Practice, Theory, and Research 37(2):34–51, 2009

Merrell KW, Gueldner BA, Ross SW, et al: How effective are school bullying intervention programs? A meta-analysis of intervention research. School Psychology Quarterly 23(1):26–42, 2008

Miller EM, Mondschein ES: Sexual harassment and bullying: similar, but not the same. What school officials need to know. Clearing House 90(5–6):191–197, 2017

Mishna F, Cook C, Gadalla T, et al: Cyber bullying behaviors among middle and high school students. Am J Orthopsychiatry 80(3):362–374, 2010 20636942

Moore SE, Norman RE, Suetani S, et al: Consequences of bullying victimization in childhood and adolescence: a systematic review and meta-analysis. World J Psychiatry 7(1):60–76, 2017 28401049

Morse v. Frederick, 551 U.S. 393, 127 S. Ct. 2618, 168 L. Ed. 2d 290 (2007)

Nansel TR, Overpeck M, Pilla RS, et al: Bullying behaviors among US youth: prevalence and association with psychosocial adjustment. JAMA 285(16):2094–2100, 2001 11311098

Newman-Carlson D, Horne AM: Bully Busters: a psychoeducational intervention for reducing bullying behavior in middle school students. J Couns Dev 82(3):259–267, 2004

Newman-Carlson D, Horne AM, Bartolomucci CL: Bully Busters: A Teacher's Manual for Helping Bullies, Victims, and Bystanders. Champaign, IL, Research Press, 2000

O'Brennan LM, Bradshaw CP, Sawyer AL: Examining developmental differences in the social-emotional problems among frequent bullies, victims, and bully/victims. Psychol Sch 46(2):100–115, 2009

Olweus D: Bullying at school: basic facts and effects of a school based intervention program. J Child Psychol Psychiatry 35(7):1171–1190, 1994 7806605

Olweus D: Bullying at school: knowledge base and an effective intervention program. Ann N Y Acad Sci 794(1):265–276, 1996

Olweus D: Bullying at school: tackling the problem. OECD Obs 225:24–26, 2001

Olweus D, Limber SP: Bullying in school: evaluation and dissemination of the Olweus Bullying Prevention Program. Am J Orthopsychiatry 80(1):124–134, 2010 20397997

Olweus D, Limber S, Mihalic SF: Bullying Prevention Program: Blueprints for Violence Prevention, Book Nine. Blueprints for Violence Prevention Series. Boulder, CO, Center for the Study and Prevention of Violence, Institute of Behavioral Science, University of Colorado, 1999

Orpinas P, Home AM, Staniszewski D: School bullying: changing the problem by changing the school. School Psych Rev 32(3):431–444, 2003

People v. Marquan, 24 N.Y.3d 1, 19 N.E.3d 480, 994 N.Y.S.2d 554 (2014)

Pepler DJ, Craig WM, Connolly J, et al: Bullying, sexual harassment, dating violence, and substance use among adolescents, in The Violence and Addiction Equation: Theoretical and Clinical Issues in Substance Abuse and Relationship Violence. Edited by Wekerle C, Wall AM. New York, Brunner-Routledge, 2002, pp 151–166

Rettew DC, Pawlowski S: Bullying. Child Adolesc Psychiatr Clin N Am 25(2):235–242, 2016 26980126

Rigby K: Peer victimisation at school and the health of secondary school students. Br J Educ Psychol 69(Pt 1):95–104, 1999 10230345

Roland E: Bullying, depressive symptoms and suicidal thoughts. Educ Res 44(1):55–67, 2002

Ryoo JH, Wang C, Swearer SM: Examination of the change in latent statuses in bullying behaviors across time. Sch Psychol Q 30(1):105–122, 2015 25111466

Salmivalli C, Kärnä A, Poskiparta E: Counteracting bullying in Finland: The KiVa program and its effect on different forms of being bullied. Int J Behav Dev 35(5):405–411, 2011

Scholte RHJ, Engels RCME, Overbeek G, et al: Stability in bullying and victimization and its association with social adjustment in childhood and adolescence. J Abnorm Child Psychol 35(2):217–228, 2007 17295065

Schwartz D, Hopmeyer Gorman A: Community violence exposure and children's academic functioning. J Educ Psychol 95(1):163–173, 2003

Seeley K, Tombari ML, Bennett LJ, et al: Bullying in Schools Bullying in Schools: An Overview. Washington, DC, Office of Justice Programs, U.S. Department of Justice, 2011. Available at: www.ojjdp.gov/pubs/234205.pdf. Accessed March 20, 2019.

Smith PK, Cowie H, Olafsson RF, et al: Definitions of bullying: a comparison of terms used, and age and gender differences, in a fourteen-country international comparison. Child Dev 73(4):1119–1133, 2002 12146737

Smokowski PR, Kopasz KH: Bullying in school: an overview of types, effects, family characteristics, and intervention strategies. Children and Schools 27(2):101–110, 2005

Spriggs AL, Iannotti RJ, Nansel TRB, et al: Adolescent bullying involvement and perceived family, peer and school relations: commonalities and differences across race/ethnicity. J Adolesc Health 41(3):283–293, 2007 17707299

Spurling RA: The Bully Free School Zone Character Education Program: A Study of Impact on Five Western North Carolina Middle Schools. Doctoral dissertation. Johnson City, East Tennessee State University, 2004. Available at: http://dc.etsu.edu/etd/939. Accessed March 20, 2019.

Srabstein JC, Berkman BE, Pyntikova E: Antibullying legislation: a public health perspective. J Adolesc Health 42(1):11–20, 2008 18155025

State v. Bishop, 787 S.E.2d 814, 368 N.C. 869 (2016)

Stein N: Bullying or sexual harassment? The missing discourse of rights in an era of zero tolerance. Ariz Law Rev 45:783–799, 2003

StopBullying.gov: Misdirections in Bullying Prevention and Intervention. Washington, DC, U.S. Department of Health and Human Services, 2017. Available at: www.stopbullying.gov/sites/default/files/2017-10/misdirections-in-prevention.pdf. Accessed March 20, 2019.

Stuart-Cassel V, Ariana MPPA, Springer BJF: Analysis of State Bullying Laws and Policies. Washington, DC, U.S. Department of Education, 2011. Available at: https://www2.ed.gov/rschstat/eval/bullying/state-bullying-laws/state-bullying-laws.pdf. Accessed March 20. 2019.

Swearer SM, Doll B: Bullying in schools: an ecological framework. Journal of Emotional Abuse 2(2–3):7–23, 2001

Swearer Napolitano SM: Risk Factors for and Outcomes of Bullying and Victimization. Educ Psychol Pap Publ 132, 2011. Available at: http://digitalcommons.unl.edu/edpsychpapers/132. Accessed March 20, 2019.

Swearer SM, Song SY, Cary PT, et al: Psychosocial correlates in bullying and victimization. Journal of Emotional Abuse 2(2–3):95–121, 2001

Takizawa R, Maughan B, Arseneault L: Adult health outcomes of childhood bullying victimization: evidence from a five-decade longitudinal British birth cohort. Am J Psychiatry 171(7):777–784, 2014 24743774

Taylor CA, Liang B, Tracy AJ, et al: Gender differences in middle school adjustment, physical fighting, and social skills: evaluation of a social competency program. J Prim Prev 23(2):259–272, 2002

Thornton TN, Carole Craft Linda L, Dahlberg MA, et al: Best Practices of Youth Violence Prevention: A Sourcebook for Community Action. Atlanta, GA, Centers for Disease Control and Prevention, 2002

Tinker v. Des Moines Independent Community School District 393 U.S. 503 1969

Tippett N, Wolke D: Socioeconomic status and bullying: a meta-analysis. Am J Public Health 104(6):e48–e59, 2014 24825231

Ttofi MM, Farrington DP, Ttofi MM, et al: Effectiveness of school-based programs to reduce bullying: a systematic and meta-analytic review. J Exp Criminol 7:27–56, 2011

U.S. Department of Education: Student Reports for Bullying: Results From the 2015 School Crime Supplement to the National Crime Victimization Survey. Washington, DC, U.S. Department of Education, 2016. Retrieved from https://nces.ed.gov/pubs2017/2017015.pdf. Accessed March 20, 2019.

van der Wal MF, de Wit CAM, Hirasing RA: Psychosocial health among young victims and offenders of direct and indirect bullying. Pediatrics 111(6 Pt 1):1312–1317, 2003 12777546

Van Schoiack-Edstrom L, Frey KS, Beland K: Changing adolescents' attitudes about relational and physical aggression: an early evaluation of a school-based intervention. School Psychology Review 31(2):201–216, 2002

Vazsonyi A, Powell G, Lamb-Parker F, et al: Impact of PeaceBuilders Violence Prevention Approach on Self-Reported Bullying Perpetration with Elementary School-Age Girls. Long Beach, CA, PeaceBuilders, n.d. Available at: www.peacebuilders.com/media/pdfs/research/BullyBrief.pdf. Accessed March 20, 2019.

Wang J, Iannotti RJ, Nansel TR: School bullying among adolescents in the United States: physical, verbal, relational, and cyber. J Adolesc Health 45(4):368–375, 2009 19766941

White A, Raczynski K, Pack C, et al: Evaluation Report: The Safe School Ambassadors Program: A Student Led Approach to Reducing Mistreatment and Bullying in Schools. Santa Rosa, CA, Community Matters, 2011. Available at: http://community-matters.org/downloads/EvaluationReportSSA2011.pdf. Accessed March 20. 2019.

Williams KR, Guerra NG: Prevalence and predictors of Internet bullying. J Adolesc Health 41(6)(suppl 1):S14–S21, 2007 18047941

Wolke D, Woods S, Stanford K, et al: Bullying and victimization of primary school children in England and Germany: prevalence and school factors. Br J Psychol 92(Pt 4):673–696, 2001 11762868

Zarghami M: Selection of person of the year from public health perspective: promotion of mass clusters of copycat self-immolation. Iran J Psychiatry Behav Sci 6(1):1–11, 2012 24644463

Zenere FJ 3rd, Lazarus PJ: The decline of youth suicidal behavior in an urban, multicultural public school system following the introduction of a suicide prevention and intervention program. Suicide Life Threat Behav 27(4):387–402, 1997 9444734

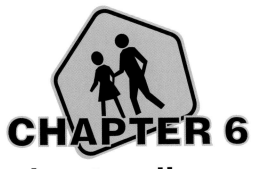

CHAPTER 6

Understanding and Addressing Youth Sexual Violence

Sophie Rosseel, M.D.

Anne B. McBride, M.D.

Michael B. Kelly, M.D.

A child's life is like a piece of paper on which every person leaves a mark.

Chinese proverb

Case Vignette

Julia is a 16-year-old girl referred to her school counselor after she had a "breakdown" in her second-period class. Julia's teacher became especially concerned after observing multiple superficial cuts on her left forearm, mostly covered by her long-sleeve blouse. As Julia talks with her school counselor, she reports that she has been experiencing increasing thoughts of suicide. Julia states that she has been feeling sad and hopeless over the past month, and last night she contemplated "ending it all" by taking an overdose of the sleeping pills she knew were in her mother's bathroom. She says that there have been times over the past month when she felt so overwhelmed by sadness that she cut herself.

The school counselor alerts the school resource officer that Julia will need an emergent psychiatric evaluation and possible inpatient hospitalization given the danger she poses to herself.

Julia begins to cry again while waiting for the resource officer to arrive. She tells the counselor that her suicidal thoughts began after an incident that occurred last month with another student, Bryan, the 17-year-old boyfriend of her good friend, Charlotte. Julia states that about 2 months ago, she was at a party with Bryan while Charlotte was home sick. She says that she and Bryan became intoxicated with alcohol and had consensual sex. Julia notes that she felt extremely guilty after the incident, and she ignored Bryan's text messages to her following the incident. She tried to avoid Bryan at school, but about a month ago, she agreed to talk to him on campus. Julia says that Bryan insisted they talk "somewhere private" so that Charlotte would not see them talking. She agreed to go into an empty storage closet to talk with him. Bryan told her that he wanted to have sex again, but she told him no. She says he began kissing her despite her requests for him to stop. Julia adds that Bryan continued kissing her, forced her to the ground, and "we had sex again." She reports that she refused Bryan's advances and that the incident felt "wrong"; however, she felt uncertain whether Bryan had raped her because she had previously consented to having sex with him. Julia discloses to the school counselor that she ultimately told Charlotte what happened, but Charlotte did not believe that Bryan forced her into sexual activity and then began harassing Julia on social media by calling her a "slut." Julia reveals that she has been too ashamed to tell her parents, became more and more depressed, and recently began contemplating suicide.

The school resource officer determines that Julia meets criteria for an emergency psychiatric hold, and she is transported to the community mental health crisis center. The resource officer returns to campus, speaks to the school counselor, and learns that Julia described being the victim of a sexual assault on campus a month ago. The officer accesses Bryan's previous legal history and learns that he had been accused of sexual assault once in the past, but the matter was not adjudicated. The officer contacts Bryan, informs him of his rights, and obtains a statement from him. Bryan reports that he did engage in consensual sexual intercourse on two occasions with Julia, including one incident that occurred on campus. He admits that during the second incident, he may have "gone too far," and although Julia told him she did not want to have sex, "her body was saying yes." Bryan was taken into custody and charged with sexual assault.

In this chapter, we aim to examine youth sexual violence and the mechanisms, behaviors, and correlates of youth sexual offending. A background of juvenile sexual violence and juvenile stalking can be found in Chapter 3, "Inconvenient Truths," and in this chapter we aim to provide further research on additional juvenile sexual offenses and sexual behaviors and to provide practical considerations regarding sexual violence on school campus.

Youth Sexual Consent

Consent is perhaps the most critical and fundamental issue in understanding the topic of sexual violence. At its basis, sexual violence in all forms assumes a lack of mutual sexual consent between two individuals. Sexual consent capacity in adults is met if "the requisite rationality, knowledge, and voluntariness are present"; however, the topic of sexual consent becomes significantly more complex if the involved parties are below the age of consent (California Senate 2014, p. 5; Lyden 2007). California Bill SB 967 amended the California education code to mandate updated sexual assault policies in postsecondary schools receiving public funds. Sexual consent now requires "affirmative, conscious, and voluntary agreement to engage in sexual activity" (California Senate 2014, Section 1).

Adolescence is marked by a period of rapid physiological, psychological, and sexual maturation. Sexual expression is a common and normative part of adolescent development into adulthood. For example, a Kaiser Family Foundation survey regarding youth sexual experiences found that 56% of teenagers ages 15–17 had been intimate or sexual with someone, and 37% had had sexual intercourse (Hoff et al. 2003). However, reports of lack of mutual consent in adolescent sexual experiences are not uncommon. The same Kaiser Family Foundation survey found that 29% of teenagers ages 15–17 reported feeling "a lot" or "some" pressure to have sex, with 59% agreeing with the statement that there is pressure to have sex by a certain age (Hoff et al. 2003). Furthermore, 24% of teenagers ages 15–17 reported having a sexual experience they did not really want to have, and 33% reported being involved in a relationship they felt was moving too fast sexually. These statistics bolster the assertion made by Drobac (2006) regarding the voluntariness of sexual consent among adolescents that "acquiescence does not necessarily equate to consent" (p. 37). This information raises the question: which criteria must be satisfied before sexual consent capacity in youth is reached?

With regard to age of sexual consent, laws are aimed at balancing adolescent sexual freedom and expression with concurrent protection from statutory rape and adult predation. Kourany et al. (1986, p. 171) wrote that theoretical age of sexual consent "should not be so early that little protection is provided for a child. Conversely, it should not be so late that a [person] can be held for statutory rape when the 'victim' is fully capable of informed consent and readily acquiesced to a proposal or even invited a sexual relationship." In the United States, where the age of sexual consent is state dependent, legal age varies between 16 and 18 years, with varied close-in-age exemptions. In our view, the discrepancy in statewide laws and lack of expert consensus attests to the lack of clarity for which criteria define adolescent sexual consent.

guidelines on preventing and responding to sexual harassment (Tables 6–1 and 6–2). Foremost, schools receiving public funds must enforce Title IX of the Education Amendments of 1972, which aims to prevent discrimination in schools on the basis of gender. Specifically, Title IX prohibits both quid pro quo and hostile environment types of sexual harassment in schools and enforces the appointment of a Title IX coordinator within schools (Hill and Kearl 2011).

Campus Sexual Assault

Definition and Prevalence

Sexual assault can be defined as "a more inclusive term that covers a range of sex acts, including physically forced sexual contact (e.g., kissing or touching), verbally coerced intercourse, and any acts that constitute rape" (Abbey and McAuslan 2004, p. 747). Youth sexual assault and campus sexual assault recently have gained particular media attention. Current studies of college women report rates of completed rape between 0.5% and 8.4%, rates of attempted rape between 1.1% and 3.8%, and rates of unwanted sexual contact between 1.8% and 34% (Fedina et al. 2018). One study wherein only male college students were interviewed reported that 15% had forced intercourse with a woman (Rapaport and Burkhart 1984).

Assault Perpetration Models

Multiple characteristics have been associated with youth offenders of sexual assault and sexually coercive behavior. Personality and attitudinal characteristics associated with immaturity, irresponsibility, sexual aggression, and lack of social conscience were found to be predictive of sexually coercive behavior among college males (Rapaport and Burkhart 1984). Some research has shown that fraternity members were more likely to commit both verbal coercion and physical force as a sexually coercive method (Tyler et al. 1998), and perceived high-risk fraternities had higher levels of sexual aggression, hostility toward females, and peer support for sexual assault compared with perceived low-risk fraternities (Humphrey and Kahn 2000).

Hostile gender beliefs and callous attitudes in youth perpetrators have demonstrated relevance in campus sexual assault. In a study conducted by Abbey and McAuslan (2004), 35% of male college students reported perpetrating at least one sexual assault (described as forced sexual contact, verbal sexual coercion, or attempted or completed rape) since age 14. Following a 1-year time interval, participants were resurveyed, and 14% of the same group reported perpetrating sexual assault within that 1 year. Interestingly, on further subgroup delineation, 59% of men were classified as

TABLE 6–1. Tips for preventing sexual harassment at school

Enforce Title IX and appoint an official school Title IX coordinator to handle sexual harassment policies and complaints.

Adopt an official school sexual harassment policy and widely distribute the policy to students and parents.

Plan a school assembly on sexual harassment.

Provide training to staff on protocols to follow when reports of sexual harassment are made.

Source. Adapted from Hill and Kearl (2011).

TABLE 6–2. How to respond to sexual harassment at school

If sexual harassment is observed by an educator, state the behavior and stop the behavior.

Send the harasser to the principal or guidance counselor and notify the harasser's parents.

Use the incident as a platform for education about sexual harassment.

When a student reports sexual harassment, listen carefully and nonjudgmentally. Encourage the student to write down the incident in detail and offer the student information about his or her rights.

Assist the student in reporting the incident if he or she chooses to.

Source. Adapted from Hill and Kearl (2011).

nonassaulters (no offenses at either time point), 26% were past assaulters (offense prior to first time point), 6% were new assaulters (offense between first and second time point), and 9% were repeat assaulters (offenses at both time points). Comparing past assaulters with repeat assaulters, repeat assaulters demonstrated greater hostile gender role beliefs, callous attitudes, and adolescent delinquency, leading the authors to hypothesize that "extreme attitudes" may persist in the repeat assaulters and contribute more critically to offending (Abbey and McAuslan 2004). Interestingly, the data also indicated that the majority of offenders began offending during adolescence, and a large proportion of previously offending adolescents stopped offending (Abbey and McAuslan 2004). This evidence is similarly supported by Seto and Barbaree's (1997) developmental course for perpetrators, proposing "one course…characterized by an early onset of sexual activity and delinquency that continues into adulthood, and the second course…characterized by a more short-term opportunistic approach that desists after adolescence" (cited in Abbey and McAuslan 2004, p. 748).

In terms of the psychological development of a sexual assault perpetrator, Malamuth et al. (1991) postulated contributions from two independent mechanisms leading to sexual offending: hostile masculine attitudes and sexual promiscuity. The model of Malamuth and colleagues first approaches coercion from biological, psychological, and environmental influences as a needs-based approach learned from childhood experiences through association with delinquent peer groups as well as through general cultural attitudes toward coercion. Second, the model approaches sexual promiscuity as a form of expression of power and maintenance of self-esteem. The research of Malamuth and colleagues demonstrated that the combination of hostile attitudes and sexual promiscuity leads to sexual aggression, and particularly that "when those with higher levels of hostile masculinity engage in promiscuous sex, it is more likely to be coercive, compared with those relatively low on hostile masculinity" (Malamuth et al. 1991, p. 680).

Campus-Wide Prevention Approaches

The prevalence and seriousness of campus sexual assault has resulted in widespread educational programming targeting sexual assault prevention. A meta-analysis conducted by Anderson and Whiston (2005) analyzed 69 studies assessing effectiveness of college sexual assault education programs. Their research demonstrated the greatest effect sizes with rape knowledge and rape attitudes on quantitative measures, indicating that educational programs led to the greatest positive change in these categories. Statistical significance was also found with programming in behavioral intentions, rape-related attitudes, and incidence of sexual assault, although the effect sizes for these areas were likely clinically insignificant. Last, no statistical significance was found with educational programming on rape empathy or rape behaviors. Importantly, the interventional styles that were most effective on attitudes were those that concentrated on gender-role socialization, general information about rape, rape myths and facts, and risk-reduction strategies. In-depth, focused programming was found to be more effective than superficial programming, and professional presenters were superior to graduate student or peer presenters (Anderson and Whiston 2005).

Youth Dating Violence, Youth Date Rape, and Drug-Facilitated Sexual Assault

Youth dating violence is considered a public health concern with severe physical and mental health consequences (Vagi et al. 2013). Rates of intimate partner violence in adolescents range from 15% to 40% (Rickert et al. 2002). A review by Vagi et al. (2013) outlined numerous correlates of dating violence perpetration, including depression, general aggression, prior dating violence, parental marital conflict, and engagement in peer violence. In another study, predictors of female dating violence perpetration included having friends who were victims of dating violence, using alcohol, and being of a race other than white; in contrast, adolescent male perpetration predictors included attitudes accepting of dating violence (Foshee et al. 2001).

Date rape can be defined as unwanted, forced sexual intercourse between two intimate partners. In contrast, when unwanted, nonmutual intercourse occurs between individuals who know each other but are not romantically involved, this is termed *acquaintance rape.* When the perpetrator is completely unknown to the victim, this is termed *stranger rape.* When the influence of drugs or other psychoactive substances is used to facilitate rape, usually to pacify the victim during the commission of the assault, this is referred to as *drug-facilitated sexual assault* (DFSA).

The prevalence of date rape in adolescents varies widely in research studies from 20% to 68%, with slightly lower rates found in college-age women (Rickert and Wiemann 1998). Exact prevalence of youth date rape is difficult to ascertain because of concern about underreporting, which is particularly problematic in youth, as well as the fact that when date rape occurs, "the victim and the perpetrator usually view the occurrence of sexual assault very differently, wherein the woman usually feels as if she has been victimized, whereas the perpetrator perceives that no harm has been done" (Rickert and Wiemann 1998, p. 167, citing Parrot and Bechhofer 1991).

Rickert and Wiemann (1998) outlined four theoretical models of date and acquaintance rape perpetration: 1) psychiatric and psychological, related to individual characteristics of the victim and perpetrator, 2) cultural norms of violence and sexism, related to expectation of sexual violence in masculine roles, 3) social context, related to integration of social behavioral components, and 4) developmental, related to "intergenerational transmission" of sexual violence.

DFSA is a subset of date rape and acquaintance rape particularly prevalent among college students. Multiple substances have been implicated in DFSA, including alcohol, marijuana, benzodiazepines such as flunitrazepam (Rohypnol), gamma hydroxybutyric acid, cocaine, and amphetamines. Substances can be ingested voluntarily or involuntarily without the victim's knowledge, rendering the victim both incapacitated and unable to provide sexual consent. The prevalence of certain and suspected drug-facilitated assault with involuntary incapacitation is 0.6% and 1.7%, respectively, in female college students, and 7.8% with voluntary incapacitation (Krebs et al. 2007). Of male college sexual assault perpetrators of incapacitated sexual assault, 81% of offenders reported drinking alcohol prior to the assault, and none of the offenders considered the assault to be rape (Krebs et al. 2007).

Strong contributors to the continued perpetration of youth date rape are rape myths and gender-bound stereotypes particularly ingrained in youth. *Rape myths* can be defined as "false beliefs used…to shift the blame of rape from perpetrators to victims" (Suarez and Gadalla 2010, p. 2010). Incorrect ideas or cognitive distortions regarding female sexuality and the victim's personal culpability strongly influence the perception of date rape, specifically in terms of negative attitudes toward rape victims as well as the traditionality of gender roles (Muehlenhard and MacNaughton 1988). Greater acceptance of rape myths has been associated with a number of factors, including male gender, lower educational levels, sexual aggression, sexual coercion, elite athlete status, sexist attitudes toward women, and other discriminatory attitudes (Suarez and Gadalla 2010). Differences between genders in attributing responsibility of rape have led to the recommendation of gender-specific rape education (Cowan and Campbell 1995).

Schools can assist in prevention of adolescent dating violence. Research attests to the effectiveness of school-based prevention programs (Table 6–3). A systematic review by De Koker et al. (2014) examined six randomized controlled trials of community and school interventions, three of which demonstrated positive results in prevention of perpetration or victimization in adolescent intimate partner violence. More effective programs were longer in duration, were more comprehensive, had individual-level curricula, and included community-based elements.

Social Media Violence: Sexting and Digital Dating Abuse

Increasing prevalence and accessibility of social media, the Internet, and cellular phones have led to new mechanisms of sexual violence among youth. Given the recency of widespread online communication, significant research is ongoing regarding the prevalence, legal implications, and psychological effects of the distribution of sexually explicit content and online-mediated sexual violence.

Scope and Prevalence

Digital dating abuse (DDA) can generally be defined as "the use of digital media to monitor, control, threaten, harass, pressure, or coerce a dating partner" (Reed et al. 2017, p. 79). The prevalence of overall digital sexual coercion, overall digital direct aggression, and overall digital monitoring or control in high school students' relationships has been found

TABLE 6–3. **Tips for dating abuse prevention programming**

Tailor programming to the specific audience, namely, age, race/ethnicity, and gender

Older adolescents may benefit from more focus on dating relationships, whereas younger adolescents may benefit from general conflict resolution and communication

Address gender stereotypes and traditional gender roles

Encourage and build youth attitudes that refuse to accept dating violence

Support healthy and considerate youth relationships

Encourage skill building for bystanders

Implement peer educators and peer counselors to assist in promoting a safe school environment

Source. Adapted from Noonan and Charles (2009).

to be remarkably high: 32%, 46%, and 54%, respectively (Reed et al. 2017). Importantly, DDA has been significantly associated with off-line psychological aggression, which is postulated to be due to implementation of similar psychological control strategies, but it has not necessarily been associated with off-line physical aggression (Borrajo et al. 2015). With respect to teen attitudes toward DDA, adolescent males were noted to view DDA as less severe than face-to-face abuse because they found it "easier to stop and ignore"; in contrast, adolescent females found it more severe, believing that DDA presented "more opportunities for abuse" and was more intrusive (Stonard et al. 2017).

Implications and Outcomes

Sexting, the colloquial term for texting sexual content, has become a critical point of discussion with regard to youth sexual behavior. *Sexting* can be generally defined as the communication of sexually suggestive or explicit imagery via text message. In a 2011 phone survey of 1,560 youth Internet users ages 10–17 years, the prevalence of youth appearing in, creating, or receiving nude or nearly nude images was 9.6%, although other studies have reported sexting prevalence as high as 28% (Mitchell et al. 2011; Temple et al. 2012). More specifically, 5.9% of youth surveyed reported receiving a sexually explicit image, and 1% of youth reported engaging in creation or distribution of sexual imagery, which could constitute violation of child pornography laws (Mitchell et al. 2011).

A number of concerns have arisen with regard to youth sexting, including appropriate consent, privacy, psychological effects, and impact on subsequent employment or educational opportunities. With regard to consent, a study by Englander (2012) found the most frequent motivation for sexting to be pressure or coercion, and for girls, coercion motivated about half of sexting. With regard to mental health impact, one survey found that 21% of youth who were in or created images were consequently "very or extremely upset, embarrassed, or afraid" (Mitchell et al. 2011). Sexting in adolescents also has been associated with high-risk sexual and substance use behaviors, a history of being cyberbullied, and a history of being physically hurt by a significant other in the past year (Dake et al. 2012).

State legislatures are now charged with creating law that differentiates normative adolescent sexual behavior from exploitive and explicit material involving minors. The Third National Juvenile Online Victimization Study found that law enforcement handled approximately 3,477 cases involving youth-produced sexual images during 2008 and 2009 (Walsh et al. 2013). Two-thirds of those cases involved an *aggravating* circumstance, of which approximately a third involved a minor engaging in malicious, nonconsensual, or abusive behavior. A survey found that malicious intent or bullying, distribution, large age difference, or graphic imagery were present most commonly when prosecutors decided to file charges against a minor (Walsh et al. 2013). The outcomes of sexting cases included an arrest in 36% of the aggravated youth-only cases and 18% of the nonaggravated youth-only cases.

Practical Considerations

Education about and prevention of digital dating violence should be a focus for schools and families. With technology continually changing and evolving, it can be difficult for schools and families to keep up with potential digital problems as they arise. School administrators and counselors can actively remain aware of the evolving digital landscape through updates from national professional organizations. For example, in 2017, the American Academy of Pediatrics offered tips for families when talking with children about problems such as sexting (Chassiakos 2017). Similarly, the American Academy of Child and Adolescent Psychiatry (www.aacap.org) offers "Facts for Families," which includes current, freely available information on relevant topics for children and families (e.g., "Internet Use in Children" and "Social Media and Teens"). For information on educating youth about sexting, see Table 6–4. These tips can be easily applied to school settings and used by mental health professionals, who can collaborate with families when educating students on responsible media usage. Often, parents and guardians would benefit from education from the schools and increased awareness of potential problems that come with advancing technology.

TABLE 6–4. **Tips for educating youth about sexting**

Educate youth early about sexting and digital dating abuse. If youth have unsupervised access to digital devices (e.g., cell phones, computers with Internet access), review appropriate versus inappropriate content and communication.

Discuss with youth what behaviors are considered sexting and advise them that if they receive or are asked to send sexual content, they should tell a trusted adult (e.g., parent, teacher, counselor).

Teach youth that any content they send electronically may be permanently accessible and widely distributed or shared with others.

Inform youth that sending, receiving, or requesting digital sexual content may be considered criminal behavior that is punishable by time in a detention facility.

If youth are already involved in sending, receiving, or requesting digital sexual content, discuss with them that it is never too late to tell a trusted adult, even if they feel pressured to participate in the digital exchange.

Whenever possible, monitor digital media use. If youth are spending excessive amounts of time online or communicating with others by texting, check in with them and review appropriate media use.

Set limits on access to digital devices. For example, limit use of cell phones at bedtime. Keep computers or televisions with Internet access in shared family rooms and out of youths' bedrooms.

Adults working with or supervising children and adolescents should try to stay up to date with digital media such as by periodically reviewing professional guidelines (e.g., American Academy of Pediatrics, American Academy of Child and Adolescent Psychiatry).

Overview of Youth Sexual Offenders

Categorization

Juvenile sexual offenders constitute a diverse group of individuals with complex characteristics and backgrounds. Youth commit a large portion of all sexual offenses, with estimates that 20% of all rapes and 30%–50% of child molestations are perpetrated by youth younger than 20 years (Shaw and Antia 2010). In a study of youth offenders in the state of Washington conducted by Fehrenbach et al. (1986), the most common sexual offenses committed by youth were indecent liberties (59%); rape (23%); exposure (11%); and hands-off offenses including peeping, stealing underwear, and making obscene phone calls or sending obscene letters (7%). The majority of victims of youth sexual offenders were younger than age 12, and a third of victims were family members.

Committing sexual violence during adolescence is not a normative aspect of sexual development (Fehrenbach et al. 1986). Male adolescent sexual assaulters have been shown to demonstrate moderate to severe maladjustment (84%), chronic behavioral school problems (72%), and antisocial behavior (56%) (Awad and Saunders 1991). Sexual abuse history may also play a role in increasing perpetration risk in predisposed individuals; research has demonstrated greater sexually coercive behavior in those who have been victims of sexual abuse (Ryan and Otonichar 2016).

According to research by Finkelhor et al. (2009), juveniles commit approximately one-third (35.6%) of all sexual offenses against youth. Furthermore, compared with adult sex offenders committing sexual violence against minors, youth offenders are more likely to offend at school and in groups, and the vast majority of juvenile offenders are older than 12 years, with a steep rate of rise between ages 12 and 14.

As stated in Chapter 3, there have been several efforts to classify offenders in terms of common characteristics. Such efforts include Shaw and Antia's (2010) categorization of youth sexual offenders (offenders with paraphilic disorders, offenders with antisocial traits, offenders with neurological compromise, and offenders with impaired social skills) as well as Ryan and Otonichar's (2016) categorization of youth sexual offenders (youth with paraphilic disorders, youth with conduct disorders, and youth with general psychopathology). These classifications aim to provide commonality among the diversity of offenders in the hopes of understanding common mechanisms in pathogenesis and to form targeted treatments to prevent recidivism (Ryan and Otonichar 2016). Currently, evidence reveals that juvenile offenders who have undergone treatment have reduced recidivism rates, and, in fact, juvenile sexual offenders are actually at greater risk for subsequently committing a nonsexual offense than a sexual offense (Ryan and Otonichar 2016).

Assessment

When sexual violence occurs on campus, law enforcement may become involved when the behavior constitutes a crime. Youth sex offenders who enter the juvenile justice system typically undergo formal evaluation by a mental health professional with expertise in development, juvenile justice, and sexual violence risk assessment. Performing such an assessment is beyond the scope of this book. However, many of the principles involved in conducting a risk assessment that are described in Chapter 9, "Avoiding Danger," apply to a sexual violence risk assessment. Structured assessments specific to youth sexual violence have been developed to aid in these evaluations.

Youth who have been adjudicated for a sexual offense may return to school or receive educational services in a residential facility depending on the level of risk the individual poses to other youth. Sometimes, a juvenile's probation terms will include specific supervision needs or limitations on certain individuals with whom the juvenile can associate. For example, a youth who has sexually offended against a young child may not be allowed unsupervised contact with young children. School administrators and campus resource officers may need to work closely with the youth's probation officer to understand the juvenile's specific requirements and ensure the safety of other students on campus.

Prevention

Interventions for Students

A variety of primary prevention programs aimed at reducing sexual violence among youth have been implemented around the United States with mixed results. A meta-analysis by DeGue et al. (2014) identified the following primary prevention programs designed for middle and high school students as having some evidence base for reducing sexual violence:

1. *Safe Dates* is a curriculum designed for middle school students that is composed of 10 separate 45-minute teacher-led sessions. The curriculum also includes a poster contest and a 45-minute-long student-produced play on dating violence. A randomized controlled trial by Foshee et al. (2004) concluded that eighth graders who participated in the program were less likely than the control group to be both perpetrators and victims of sexual violence. More recently, Safe Dates was adapted into a family-based teen dating abuse prevention program for 13- to 15-year-olds and was evaluated with a randomized controlled trial design (Foshee et al. 2012). Foshee and colleagues showed that only 3% of teens who underwent the family-based adaptation of Safe Dates were the victims of physical dating violence, as opposed to 11% in the control group.
2. *Shifting Boundaries* is a school-based violence prevention program designed for sixth and seventh graders (Taylor et al. 2013). The program consists of two main components. The first is composed of six sessions of classroom-based activities characterized by psychoeducation (e.g., discussion of healthy relationships, consequences for sexual violence perpetrators, and gender). The second component is building-based and involves restraining orders, increased faculty and security staff in "hot spots" for potential violence (based on student input), and posters throughout the school designed to increase awareness

and reporting in relation to violence. A randomized controlled trial was conducted with more than 2,500 New York City middle schoolers who received the classroom-based intervention, the building-based intervention, a combined intervention (i.e., both classroom and building-based), or no intervention. Taylor and colleagues found that the building-only and combined interventions reduced sexual violence involving peers or dating partners 6 months following the intervention. Furthermore, the building-only intervention was associated with reductions in sexually violent behavior by classmates. Therefore, the building-only intervention may be a particularly cost-effective intervention for schools (Taylor et al. 2013).

3. *Dating Matters* is a free online course created by the Centers for Disease Control and Prevention with the goal of providing "educators and others working with youth knowledge of teen dating violence and resources that provide evidence-based solutions to prevent primary, secondary and tertiary teen dating violence" (Dating Matters website, https://vetoviolence.cdc.gov/apps/datingmatters). The course is composed of an interactive video through which participants "follow a school administrator throughout his day as he highlights what teen dating violence is and how to prevent it through graphic novel scenarios, interactive exercises, and information gathered from leading experts."

Despite a need for more studies aimed at identifying particularly effective sexual violence prevention programs, these resources provide a good starting point for educators, school administrators, and concerned parents seeking to reduce sexual violence in schools.

Interventions for Teachers

Although it is beyond the scope of this book to address the perpetration of sexual violence by school personnel, we feel that creating safeguards to help ensure that students are not victimized by trusted adults on school grounds is an essential component of developing a healthy and safe school climate. The issue of preventing sexual violence perpetrated by school personnel is an important topic, and one for which there are limited data. For instance, according to a report released in 2014 by the U.S. Government Accountability Office, no federal agencies collect comprehensive data that would quantify the prevalence of sexual abuse by school personnel (U.S. Government Accountability Office 2014). At the time of the report, only 18 states required school districts to train staff on the awareness and prevention of sexual abuse in schools. Older data from the U.S. Department of Education (Shakeshaft 2004) show that almost 7% of children attending school in the United States experience unwanted sexual contact at school and that the perpetrator is usually a teacher or a coach. This figure jumps to 10% of kindergarten through twelfth graders when including nontouching sexual offenses. Most states require background checks for public school teachers; however, the level of scrutiny provided to persons teaching in private schools or to other school personnel varies considerably.

A recent article by Wurtele et al. (2018) outlined seven standards that can be used as an "operational framework for prevention and reduced likelihood" of educator sexual misconduct. These seven standards of practice for prevention of educator sexual misconduct are as follows:

1. Screening and selecting staff
2. Implementing formal codes of conduct
3. Ensuring safe environments
4. Establishing robust staff-student communication policies, including policies on electronic and social media use
5. Educating staff, parents, and students about child sexual abuse and its prevention
6. Monitoring and supervising all staff
7. Ensuring that students, parents, and staff have opportunities to report concerns of potential breaches of the code of conduct and are protected against retaliation (whistle-blower protection)

A user-friendly Child Sexual Abuse Prevention Evaluation Tool for Organizations based on these seven standards can be found in the appendix of Wurtele and colleagues' article.

Key Points

- Sexual violence during adolescence is not a normative aspect of sexual development.

- Youth sexual consent is a fundamental issue in understanding the topic of sexual violence. There is no national expert consensus on which criteria (e.g., age, age difference between partners, verbal communication) should apply to youth consent, and current standards are state dependent.

- Sexual harassment is prevalent in schools, with more than four-fifths of students experiencing harassment. Sexual harassment most commonly involves sexual comments, jokes, gestures, or looks. Schools should follow Title IX guidelines to promote safe school environments.

- Youth sexual assault is pervasive on campus. Attitudinal and personality characteristics, particularly hostile gender beliefs and callous attitudes, are postulated to play a role in campus sexual assault. Certain college sexual assault education programs have been found to be effective.

- Youth dating violence is a public health concern, with reported rates of intimate partner violence between 15% and 40%. Notably, substances play a large role in the perpetration of sexual assault. Rape myths and gender stereotypes strongly reinforce the perpetration of date rape.

- The expansion of social media and access to the Internet have led to new methods of sexual violence among youth. Sexting can be generally defined as the communication of sexually suggestive or explicit language or imagery over text message. Youth-produced sexual images have been prosecuted by the law, most commonly when aggravating circumstances are present.

Clinical Pearls

At a minimum, schools can follow guidelines on preventing and responding to sexual harassment. Schools receiving public funds must enforce Title IX of the Education Amendments of 1972, which aims to prevent discrimination in schools based on gender.

Research on campus-wide prevention of sexual assault has found that the interventional styles most effective on attitudes are those that concentrate on gender role socialization, general information about rape, rape myths and facts, and risk-reduction strategies. In-depth, focused programming was found to be more effective than superficial programming, and professional presenters were superior to graduate student or peer presenters.

More effective programs addressing dating violence are longer in duration, more comprehensive, have individual-level curricula, and include community-based elements.

School administrators and counselors can actively remain aware of the evolving digital landscape through updates from national professional organizations.

References

Abbey A, McAuslan P: A longitudinal examination of male college students' perpetration of sexual assault. J Consult Clin Psychol 72(5):747–756, 2004 15482033

Abbey A, McAuslan P, Ross LT: Sexual assault perpetration by college men: the role of alcohol, misperception of sexual intent, and sexual beliefs and experiences. J Soc Clin Psychol 17(2):167–195, 1998

Anderson LA, Whiston SC: Sexual assault education programs: a meta-analytic examination of their effectiveness. Psychol Women Q 29(4):374–388, 2005

Awad GA, Saunders EB: Male adolescent sexual assaulters: clinical observations. J Interpers Violence 6(4):446–460, 1991

Borrajo E, Gámez-Guadix M, Calvete E: Cyber dating abuse: prevalence, context, and relationship with offline dating aggression. Psychol Rep 116(2):565–585, 2015 25799120

California Senate Bill 967, Section 67386 of the Education Code (2014)

Chassiakos YR: Talking about sexting with your children. Itasca, IL, American Academy of Pediatrics, February 2017. Available at: www.healthy children.org/English/family-life/Media/Pages/The-New-Problem-of-Sexting.aspx. Accessed July 22, 2018.

Cowan G, Campbell RR: Rape causal attitudes among adolescents. J Sex Res 32(2):145–153, 1995

Dake JA, Price JH, Maziarz L, Ward B: Prevalence and correlates of sexting behavior in adolescents. Am J Sex Educ 7(1):1–15, 2012

DeGue S, Valle LA, Holt MK, et al: A systematic review of primary prevention strategies for sexual violence perpetration. Aggress Violent Behav 19(4):346–362, 2014 29606897

De Koker P, Mathews C, Zuch M, et al: A systematic review of interventions for preventing adolescent intimate partner violence. J Adolesc Health 54(1):3–13, 2014 24125727

Drobac JA: "Developing capacity": adolescent "consent" at work, at law, and in the sciences of the mind. Journal of Juvenile Law and Policy 10(1):1–68, 2006

Englander E: Low Risk Associated With Most Teenage Sexting: A Study of 617 18-Year-Olds. Bridgewater, MA, Massachusetts Aggression Reduction Center, 2012

Fedina L, Holmes JL, Backes BL: Campus sexual assault: a systematic review of prevalence research from 2000 to 2015. Trauma Violence Abuse 19(1):76–93, 2018 26906086

Fehrenbach PA, Smith W, Monastersky C, et al: Adolescent sexual offenders: offender and offense characteristics. Am J Orthopsychiatry 56(2):225–233, 1986 3706502

Finkelhor D, Ormrod R, Chaffin M: Juveniles Who Commit Sex Offenses Against Minors. Juvenile Justice Bulletin. Washington, DC, Office of Juvenile Justice and Delinquency Prevention, Office of Justice Programs, U.S. Department of Justice, December 2009

Foshee VA, Bauman KE, Ennett ST, et al: Assessing the long-term effects of the Safe Dates program and a booster in preventing and reducing adolescent dating violence victimization and perpetration. Am J Public Health 94(4):619–624, 2004 15054015

Foshee VA, Linder F, MacDougall JE, et al: Gender differences in the longitudinal predictors of adolescent dating violence. Prev Med 32(2):128–141, 2001 11162338

Foshee VA, McNaughton Reyes HL, Ennett ST, et al: Assessing the effects of Families for Safe Dates, a family based teen dating abuse prevention program. J Adolesc Health 51(4):349–356, 2012 22999835

Hill C, Kearl H: Crossing the Line: Sexual Harassment at School. Washington, DC, American Association of University Women, 2011

Hoff T, Greene L, Davis J: National Survey of Adolescents and Young Adults: Sexual Health Knowledge Attitudes and Experiences. San Francisco, CA, Kaiser Family Foundation, 2003

Humphrey SE, Kahn AS: Fraternities, athletic teams, and rape: importance of identification with a risky group. J Interpers Violence 15(12):1313–1322, 2000

Kourany RF, Hill RY, Hollender MH: The age of sexual consent. Bull Am Acad Psychiatry Law 14(2):171–176, 1986 3730628

Krebs CP, Lindquist CH, Warner TD, et al: The Campus Sexual Assault (CSA) Study: Final Report. Washington, DC, National Institute of Justice, U.S. Department of Justice, 2007

Lipson J: Hostile Hallways: Bullying, Teasing, and Sexual Harassment in School. Washington, DC, American Association of University Women Educational Foundation, 2001

Lyden M: Assessment of sexual consent capacity. Sex Disabil 25(1):3–20, 2007

Malamuth NM, Sockloskie RJ, Koss MP, et al: Characteristics of aggressors against women: testing a model using a national sample of college students. J Consult Clin Psychol 59(5):670–681, 1991 1955602

McMaster LE, Connolly J, Pepler D, et al: Peer to peer sexual harassment in early adolescence: a developmental perspective. Dev Psychopathol 14(1):91–105, 2002 11893096

Mitchell KJ, Finkelhor D, Jones LM, et al: Prevalence and characteristics of youth sexting: a national study. Pediatrics 129(1):13–20, 2011

Muehlenhard CL, MacNaughton JS: Women's beliefs about women who "lead men on." J Soc Clin Psychol 7(1):65–79, 1988

Noonan RK, Charles D: Developing teen dating violence prevention strategies: formative research with middle school youth. Violence Against Women 15(9):1087–1105, 2009 19675364

Parrot A, Bechhofer L (eds): Acquaintance Rape: The Hidden Crime (Wiley Series on Personality Processes, Book 157). New York, Wiley, 1991

Rapaport K, Burkhart BR: Personality and attitudinal characteristics of sexually coercive college males. J Abnorm Psychol 93(2):216–221, 1984 6725755

Reed LA, Tolman RM, Ward LM: Gender matters: experiences and consequences of digital dating abuse victimization in adolescent dating relationships. J Adolesc 59:79–89, 2017 28582653

Rickert VI, Vaughan RD, Wiemann CM: Adolescent dating violence and date rape. Curr Opin Obstet Gynecol 14(5):495–500, 2002 12401977

Rickert VI, Wiemann CM: Date rape among adolescents and young adults. J Pediatr Adolesc Gynecol 11(4):167–175, 1998 9806126

Ryan EP, Otonichar JM: Juvenile sex offenders. Curr Psychiatry Rep 18(7):67, 2016 27222141

Seto MS, Barbaree HE: Sexual aggression as antisocial behavior: a developmental model, in Handbook of Antisocial Behavior. Edited by Stoff DM, Breiling J, Maser JD. New York, Wiley, 1997, pp 524–533

Shakeshaft C: Educator Sexual Misconduct: A Synthesis of Existing Literature. Washington, DC, U.S. Department of Education, 2004

Shaw JA, Antia DK: Sexually aggressive youth, in Principles and Practice of Child and Adolescent Forensic Mental Health. Edited by Benedek E, Ash P, Scott C. Washington, DC, American Psychiatric Publishing, 2010, pp 389–402

Stonard KE, Bowen E, Walker K, et al: "They'll always find a way to get to you": technology use in adolescent romantic relationships and its role in dating violence and abuse. J Interpers Violence 32(14):2083–2117, 2017 26065711

Suarez E, Gadalla TM: Stop blaming the victim: a meta-analysis on rape myths. J Interpers Violence 25(11):2010–2035, 2010 20065313

Taylor BG, Stein ND, Mumford EA, et al: Shifting Boundaries: an experimental evaluation of a dating violence prevention program in middle schools. Prev Sci 14(1):64–76, 2013 23076726

Temple JR, Paul JA, van den Berg P, et al: Teen sexting and its association with sexual behaviors. Arch Pediatr Adolesc Med 166(9):828–833, 2012 22751805

Tillyer MS, Wilcox P, Gialopsos BM: Adolescent school-based sexual victimization: exploring the role of opportunity in a gender-specific multilevel analysis. J Crim Justice 38(5):1071–1081, 2010

Tyler K, Hoyt DR, Whitbeck LB: Coercive sexual strategies. Violence Vict 13(1):47–61, 1998 9650245

U.S. Government Accountability Office: Federal Agencies Can Better Support State Efforts to Prevent and Respond to Sexual Abuse by School Personnel. Washington, DC, Government Accountability Office, 2014

Vagi KJ, Rothman EF, Latzman NE, et al: Beyond correlates: a review of risk and protective factors for adolescent dating violence perpetration. J Youth Adolesc 42(4):633–649, 2013 23385616

Walsh W, Wolak J, Finkelhor D: Sexting: When Are State Prosecutors Deciding to Prosecute? The Third National Juvenile Online Victimization Study. Durham, NH, Crimes Against Children Research Center, 2013

Wurtele SK, Mathews B, Kenny MC: Keeping students out of harm's way: reducing risks of educator sexual misconduct. J Child Sex Abuse Jul 24:1–27, 2018 30040590 Epub ahead of print

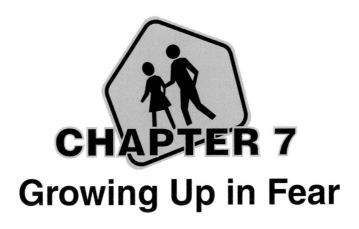

CHAPTER 7
Growing Up in Fear

School Shootings, Attacks, and Gang Violence

Tim Brennan, M.D., M.P.H.

Michael B. Kelly, M.D.

Amy Barnhorst, M.D.

Anne B. McBride, M.D.

He felt that in this crisis his laws of life were useless. Whatever he had learned of himself was here of no avail. He was an unknown quantity. He saw that he would again be obliged to experiment as he had in early youth. He must accumulate information of himself, and meanwhile he resolved to remain close upon his guard lest those qualities of which he knew nothing should everlastingly disgrace him.

Stephen Crane, The Red Badge of Courage

Case Vignette

Joshua is a 12-year-old seventh-grade boy attending a large middle school. He has a history of strong academic performance in science and math, with minor difficulties in English and history. Joshua has few friends and spends most of his free time at school alone. Joshua's mother referred him for an Individualized Education Program during grade school because of her concerns about Joshua's social skills (e.g., difficulty establishing friendships, communication deficits, problems understanding social cues), although the subsequent evaluation did not reveal any significant concerns.

Since starting middle school, Joshua has been the victim of frequent verbal taunting and occasional physical injury from a group of five male classmates. Joshua has never reported these incidents to his parents, peers, or school administrators. However, a classmate becomes alarmed after seeing a picture fall out of Joshua's math book depicting him shooting a group of boys in what appears to be a classroom.

Heartbreaking images of school children being led out of their classrooms with their hands up by law enforcement have become familiar for many Americans. Intruder drills, in which children hide under their desks and remain silent, have been added to school fire drills in preparation for an attack. Thankfully, despite how horrific they are, school mass shootings are quite rare. Using the federal government definition of mass killing as three or more people killed in a single act, no mass killings occurred in schools in the United States in 2016 and 2017 (Advanced Law Enforcement Rapid Response Training Center and Federal Bureau of Investigation 2018). However, of the 50 active shooter incidents that occurred during the same 2-year period, defined by the Federal Bureau of Investigation as "one or more individuals actively engaged in killing or attempting to kill people in a populated area" (excluding gang- and drug-related shootings), 7 incidents occurred in educational environments, leading to 5 people killed and 19 people wounded.

In fact, homicides that occur at schools are also rare. According to the most recent homicide data, from July 1, 2014 to June 30, 2015, there were 47 school-associated violent deaths (including students, staff, and nonstudents) (Musu-Gillette et al. 2018). These deaths included 28 homicides (of which 20 were students), 17 suicides, and 2 deaths due to law enforcement intervention. The 20 homicides of school-age youth (5–18 years old) that occurred at school accounted for a small fraction of the 1,168 homicides of school-age youth in total.

Other types of school violence that garner less media attention and provoke less anxiety are far more common. These include shootings with fewer victims, knifings, gang violence, and other attacks. For example, in 2016, among students ages 12–18 years, 749,400 students reported victimizations (theft and nonfatal violent victimizations) at school, and 601,300 reported victimizations away from school (Musu-Gillette et al. 2018). In 2015–2016, about 69% of schools recorded one or more violent incidents of crime (e.g., rape, sexual assault other than rape, physical attack or fight with or without a weapon, threat of physical attack with or without a weapon, robbery with or without a weapon), and 15% of schools recorded one or more serious violent incidents on campus (Musu-Gillette et al. 2018). During the 2015–2016 school year, there were 1,600 reported firearm possession incidents at school. Four percent of students ages 12–18 reported having access to a loaded gun without adult permission during the current school year. Since 1993, school violence has declined, and high schoolers reported decreased fights on school property (8%) and carrying a weapon on school property within the past 30 days (4%) in 2015. By comparison, in 1993, 12% of high school students reported being afraid of an attack or harm at school, but in 2015, only 3% of high school students endorsed such a fear (Musu-Gillette et al. 2018). In this chapter, we explore the existing literature and recommendations surrounding the prevention of and immediate and long-term (legacy) responses to school shootings and other forms of violence such as gang violence.

School Shootings and Their Aftermath

As has been the mantra of this book, prevention is the most important component of any school's approach to addressing violence. What, if anything, can be done to prevent school shootings and other firearm violence perpetrated by students?

Can We Screen Students to Detect Potential Shooters?

As referenced elsewhere in this book, screening for *potentially* violent students represents a double-edged sword. Many students will be identified as perhaps having the potential for violence but in fact will never commit any violent act (false positives). Others will be misidentified as perhaps having no potential for violence but then go on to commit violence (false negatives). As discussed in later chapters, community mental health interventions, antibullying programs, and ready access to school-based mental health services are reasonable approaches to reducing the likelihood of school violence in general. However, in the haystack that is the entire population of American schoolchildren, is it even possible to identify who is most likely to be the needle? Briefly put, there is no profile in existence that can be used to reliably identify perpetrators of targeted school violence, much less school shooters (Vossekuil et al. 2002). Thus, screening for potential school shooters among the student body is likely to be a fruitless endeavor plagued by false positives and wasted resources.

What Can Be Done to Mitigate Risk?

As school shootings have continued around the country, numerous school districts, municipalities, and states have developed crisis response plans to better prepare themselves for responding to violence on campus. The most comprehensive document to date was published by the International Association of Chiefs of Police (IACP) in collaboration with the Bureau of Justice Assistance, a component of the Department of Justice (International Association of Chiefs of Police and Bureau of Justice Assistance 2009). Reducing the potential for harm associated with school-based violence, including shootings, inevitably involves collaboration with law enforcement. School resource officers (SROs) have proliferated around the country and involve dedicated law enforcement personnel stationed at or nearby the school for the majority of their duty hours. Indeed, since 1991 there has been a National Association of School Resource Officers (NASRO), which defines school-based policing as a triad of responsibilities: teacher, informal counselor, and law enforcement officer (National Association of School Resource Officers 2018). According to a recent survey by the U.S. Department of Education, 77% of schools with more than 1,000 enrolled students had one or more SROs present once per week, 47% of schools with 500–599 students had an SRO, and 24% of schools with fewer than 300 students had an SRO (Diliberti et al. 2017).

The installation of metal detectors is another intervention that has gained popularity in many American schools and school districts. In 2011, Hankin and colleagues published a paper examining the findings from multiple studies related to the efficacy of metal detectors (Hankin et al. 2011). They concluded that there is insufficient evidence to suggest that the presence of metal detectors results in reduced violent behavior among students. One imagines that determined shooters intent on rampage would not be deterred by the presence of a metal detector on the day that they decide to commit their act.

Modifications to the physical environment of schools has also been discussed widely as a means to mitigate risk related to school violence. In 1971, C. Ray Jeffrey, a criminologist, created the approach referred to as *crime prevention through environmental design* (CPTED; Centers for Disease Control and Prevention 2018). According to the Centers for Disease Control and Prevention (2018), the following principles of CPTED can be adapted to schools:

1. Natural surveillance—maximizing visibility, particularly at entrances
2. Access management—use of landscaping and design to limit access to sensitive areas
3. Territoriality—creation of a warm and welcoming environment
4. Physical maintenance—general upkeep so as to encourage a safe environment
5. Order maintenance—clear and obvious responses to unacceptable behavior to foster a culture of accountability

Studies continue as to whether or not CPTED can lead to decreased school violence. According to the survey, the two most common factors that were reported to most limit educators' efforts to reduce or prevent crime were lack of programs for disruptive students and inadequate funding (Centers for Disease Control and Prevention 2018).

Can Active Shooter Drills Prevent Students From Being Harmed?

In 2017, the Department of Education published a report titled *Crime, Violence, Discipline, and Safety in U.S. Public Schools: Findings From the School Survey on Crime and Safety: 2015–2016* (Diliberti et al. 2017). The survey found that 74% of schools in the suburbs and 73% of schools in cities reported a formal program designed to prevent or reduce violence, compared with just 62% of schools in towns and 51% of schools in rural areas. Ninety-five percent of all schools had conducted lockdown drills, 92% of all schools had conducted evacuation procedures, and 76% of all schools had conducted shelter-in-place procedures.

The National Association of School Psychologists (NASP) and NASRO released a report in 2014 called *Best Practice Considerations for Schools in Active Shooter and Other Armed Assailant Drills*. The report, which was updated in 2017, provides a lot of helpful information for schools on how to approach this sensitive topic (National Association of School Psychologists and National Association of School Resource Officers 2014, 2017). The report cites research showing that disaster response drills "increase the probability of adaptive behavior during a crisis" (Jones and Randall 1994; Miltenberger et al. 2005, as cited in National Association of School Psychologists and National Association of School Resource Officers 2017). The report also cites research by Zhe and Nickerson (2007) involving 74 students in fourth through sixth grades who were randomly assigned to participate in a school intruder training and subsequent drill versus a control condition. The students who participated in the training and drill acquired skills for safely relocating during a school intruder event, and the training did not foster anxiety or concerns about school safety. Despite good intentions and a modicum of encouraging data, there is no empirical research supporting or refuting the potential benefits of active shooter drills (National Association of School Psychologists and National Association of School Resource Officers 2017).

The most recent NASP/NASRO report indicated that most schools' responses to armed intruders have focused on school lockdown, with recent discussion focusing on *options-based approaches*, otherwise known as "run, hide, fight." The groups recommended that school lockdowns "remain the foundation of an options-based approach to active assailant training, which allows participants to make independent decisions in evolving situations" (National Association of School Psychologists and National Association of School Resource Officers 2017, p. 1). NASP and NASRO also recommended that drills be tailored to students' developmental levels, especially when considering the use of props (e.g., airsoft guns). We are wary of using props such as airsoft guns during active shooter drills, especially when considering the potential for re-traumatizing youth who have been, or have family members who have been, victims of gun violence. School staff should also monitor students throughout the drills, paying careful attention to signs of trauma stemming from the exercise. Additional considerations and steps for implementing best practices during active shooter and other armed-assailant drills can be found on the NASP website at www.nasponline.org.

What Role Does the Mental Health System Play With Potential School Shooters?

After any mass shooting, the media and the public often respond with inquiries into the shooter's mental health history. This reinforces the perception that mental illness is a root cause of mass school shootings and that the mental health system should serve as a mechanism to identify and treat potential mass shooters before they act, as well as restrict their access to firearms. However, the reality of these propositions is far more complicated than it initially sounds.

Some public mass shooters have had histories of psychosis or other serious mental illnesses, although the level to which their psychiatric symptoms directly contributed to their violence may not be clear. Young men driven by delusions are the exception; the majority of school mass shooters do not have a confirmed history of a serious mental illness diagnosed prior to the shooting (Fox and Fridel 2016). However, many of them have in their histories referrals to or contact with mental health professionals, although many were unwilling to engage in care or take medications. Many exhibited symptoms of depression, anxiety, and suicidality (Stone 2015; Vossekuil et al. 2002). The prevalence of autism spectrum disorders among mass shooters has been found to be higher than the prevalence in the general population (Allely et al. 2017), reflecting the social deficits that may contribute to these individuals' marginalization (real or perceived) by their peers. However, research does not support that autism spectrum disorder is the cause of such violence. More importantly, if we can identify students who are struggling with social isolation or who have unmet mental health needs, they can be referred for appropriate services to address any potential risk factors associated with violence.

A common stereotype of the mass school shooter is that of a socially awkward, isolated, and resentful teen boy or young man. Knoll (2010a, 2010b) proposed a model characterizing "pseudocommando" mass murderers as angry, resentful, and socially isolated men with narcissistic and paranoid personality traits. Although Knoll's model may apply to some mass school shooters (Neuman et al. 2015), research has not revealed a reliable profile. For example, in a study of 37 incidents of targeted school violence (Vossekuil et al. 2002), only 34% of attackers were considered "loners"; 44% of attackers were involved in organized social activities. Further, 63% of attackers were perceived as being relatively easy to get along with.

Retrospective analysis has also shown that most mass school shooters reveal warning signs of their future attacks (O'Toole 2000; Vossekuil et al. 2002). As discussed in Chapter 3, "Inconvenient Truths," *leakage* leading up to the event (e.g., descriptions of violent fantasies, posting veiled threats on social media, insinuating to peers that violence is on the horizon) is common. However, there is currently no specific variable or combination of variables that reliably predicts who will become a mass school shooter. The overwhelming majority of young people who are socially isolated, resentful of peers, and/or spend a lot of time playing violent video games will never commit major acts of violence (Ash 2016). Leakage serves as a preview of their plans; these students often foretell what is to come by writing violent stories, posting veiled threats on social media, or hinting to other students about their intentions. However, regardless of the strength of these commonalities, they do not serve as reliable predictors of who will become a school shooter. Isolated loners who feel left out of the high school social milieu and write violent stories or engage in violent video games comprise a large group of people, most of whom will never commit acts of violence (Ash 2016).

Any mental illness in this group is inherently of low enough severity to allow for them to plan out their revenge fantasy, acquire weapons and ammunition, and enact their plans undetected. They are relatively high functioning and therefore are unlikely to come to the attention of the involuntary mental health system unless brought in on a dangerousness hold for making specific threats. However, most states' involuntary hold criteria specify that in order to be involuntarily committed for dangerousness, that dangerousness must be due to a mental illness. Threats of violence against peers for intimidation and revenge would not qualify. In addition, even if these individuals were admitted into the involuntary mental health system for further evaluation, it is unlikely that their commitment would be certified in court by the presiding judge in the absence of clear mental illness. This, combined with these youths' general reluctance to participate in voluntary treatment, makes it difficult for mental health providers to mitigate any psychiatric symptoms that might be contributing to their plans.

What Can Be Done to Restrict Access to Firearms?

Although it may be difficult to get potential school shooters into treatment, the mental health system might be a pathway for these individuals to be disqualified from purchasing guns. Federal law prohibits people who have ever been "committed to a mental institution" from buying a firearm from a federally licensed dealer (Gun Control Act of 1968). Mental health diagnoses, outpatient visits, and emergency holds do not meet the threshold for prohibition; only once a judge has certified the involuntary commitment in court is the patient's name submitted to the federal background check database. If a prohibited person later tries to purchase a gun from a federally licensed dealer, the dealer will run the person's name through the federal background check database, see that he or she is prohibited, and stop the sale. However, in most states, private-party sales do not require a background check, so a prohibited person could still purchase a gun from a private party or at a gun show. Future state legislation requiring that all firearm purchases include a background check and ensuring that complete records are uploaded to the National Instant Criminal Background Check System are vital steps in keeping guns out of the hands of dangerous people.

However, although some potential school shooters might be prevented from buying guns if they had been involuntarily committed by the mental health system, the majority of them will not make it far enough into the process to be treated or prohibited. In addition, even if a person has been newly prohibited through the mental health system, this background check process does little to address the guns or ammunition they might already own. Other laws restricting access to guns can fill some of these gaps, and making it more difficult for potential school shooters to access guns may reduce school mass shootings as well as other types of gun violence among adolescents and young adults.

Having a gun in the home increases the risk of both suicide and homicide of household members (Kellermann et al. 1992, 1993). Particularly when guns are stored unlocked in the home, they are readily accessible by other family members, regardless of legal status or age. Storing guns unloaded and locked away, with the ammunition in a separate location, makes it harder for teenagers to access them. Many states make it illegal through child access prevention laws for parents to have guns and ammunition accessible with children in the house (Giffords Law Center to Prevent Gun Violence 2018). Smart gun technology, which detects the authorized user of the gun and prevents use by others, is another method of decreasing an angry teenager's ability to access a family member's gun. (See Schaechter and Alvarez 2016 for a comprehensive overview on firearm violence, child development, and prevention.)

Age-based purchasing restrictions can prevent older teenagers and young adults from being able to buy high-capacity long guns with which they can kill a large number of people quickly. Federal law prohibits licensed dealers from selling handguns to anyone younger than 21, but for long guns (rifles and shotguns), the age limit is 18. Some states have raised the legal age for purchasing a long gun to 21 as well, making it more difficult for older adolescents to obtain high-capacity weapons. Many states also limit the number of guns or ammunition a person can purchase in a specific amount of time (Giffords Law Center to Prevent Gun Violence 2018).

When potential school shooters ignite concern among those around them and they may already have begun to acquire guns, extreme risk protection laws (also known as *red flag laws* or *gun violence restraining orders*) provide a unique tool to legally remove guns from their possession temporarily and prevent them from buying more. The enactment of these statutes does not require any criminal act to have taken place, nor is any mental health history or diagnosis required. Availability and details of such laws vary by state. Family members or law enforcement who are concerned about a person's risk of violence (or suicide) can petition a court to have the person's guns removed from his or her possession and for the individual to be prohibited from purchasing any guns for some time into the future. Emergency orders can be obtained quickly by law enforcement, but due process protections are in place. Respondents have the opportunity to plead their case in front of the judge within a few weeks of the initial order, and if the judge determines they are not at risk, the guns can be returned. If not, the order can be extended for up to 1 year (Frattaroli et al. 2015).

As of 2018, 14 states have passed such a law, many in response to mass shootings in which multiple people expressed concern about the person's violence potential but there was no legal recourse to prohibit the individual from legally owning or purchasing guns. In California, where such a law was passed in 2016 in the wake of the Isla Vista shooting, it has already been used to prevent workplace shootings, terrorist attacks, and school shootings.

Case Vignette *(continued)*

When the vice principal attempts to speak with Joshua about his drawing, he looks away and refuses to respond to questions. Joshua's parents and local law enforcement are notified about the drawing. Joshua and his parents reveal that he has a long-standing fascination with firearms and that he spends hours watching people play violent video games on YouTube. In addition, Joshua's father is a hunter, and the two of them enjoy practicing target shooting on Joshua's grandfather's rural property on the weekends.

Joshua ultimately agrees to speak with the school counselor. After gathering information from Joshua, his parents, and teachers, the counselor is able to deduce that Joshua has been socially isolated and bullied since entering junior high. Joshua tells the counselor that he has been thinking about ways to shoot five male classmates at school, although he does not have a day and time planned. He states that he will likely not go forward with his plan "now that everyone already knows" that he had been considering shooting some of his peers. The counselor suspects that Joshua may have an underlying autism spectrum disorder that has gone undiagnosed because of his strong academic performance and lack of behavior problems at school. The counselor performs a risk assessment for Joshua, which is outlined in Table 7–1.

Responding to Active Shooting

Immediate Response

Many Americans have become numb to the image of law enforcement officers descending on a school with their guns drawn as students file out with their hands up. The IACP guide identifies the following components of the immediate response (International Association of Chiefs of Police and Bureau of Justice Assistance 2009):

1. Get students out of harm's way via either lockdown or evacuation.
2. Use doors that lock from the inside; evacuate only if the location of the shooter is known.
3. Assess for injury and take appropriate measures.
4. Activate 911 or other emergency response.
5. Activate silent alarms if available.
6. Send students for help only if absolutely necessary.
7. Involve the school's crisis management team.
8. Begin the "calling tree" to alert parents.
9. Remain with students until told by authorities what to do.

The IACP guide calls for formal "critical incident stress debriefing" to be conducted within 24–72 hours after a serious act of violence. However, a Cochrane review by Rose et al. (2002) concluded that there is no evidence that debriefing is useful for the prevention of posttraumatic stress disorder.

Finally, the IACP guide also calls for the creation of safe, quiet spaces in schools in the aftermath of a violent event to allow students a place to reflect in a serene environment. Memorials and funerals typically involve not only the school community but the broad community at large (International Association of Chiefs of Police and Bureau of Justice Assistance 2009).

TABLE 7–1. **Risk assessment and intervention plan for Joshua**

Risk factor	Plan
Imminent danger to others	Restrict access to all firearms. Joshua's parents and grandparents should ensure that all firearms and ammunition will be locked in separate gun safes for which Joshua does not have the combination. Notify the parents of the boys Joshua was fantasizing about shooting, alerting them to the bullying that Joshua has endured in the process. The parents should agree to speak with their sons and attend a meeting at the school with Joshua's parents.
Mental health symptoms	Schedule a full psychiatric evaluation to determine a mental health diagnosis and treatment plan (e.g., level of community mental health services needed, psychotropic medication, therapy). Insist that Joshua's evaluation include someone with experience in conducting formal evaluations for autism spectrum disorder.
Social isolation	Refer Joshua to a local communication skills group that is designed for teens with pragmatic social difficulties. Encourage Joshua's parents to find outlets for their son that capitalize on his interest in electronics (e.g., computer programming lessons, participation in a local youth robotics team). Replace or limit Joshua's restrictive interests in Internet media sites and improve electronic supervision.
Ongoing violence	Place Joshua on a temporary leave from school. Request a formal risk assessment by a qualified mental health evaluator, including use of appropriate risk assessment instruments.
Access to firearms	If Joshua were involuntarily committed through the mental health system, he would be legally prohibited in most states from buying a gun from a licensed dealer but not necessarily from a private party. A gun violence restraining order or extreme risk protection order (if available in that state) would allow law enforcement to remove any guns Joshua already did own and prevent him from legally buying new ones. Discuss with Joshua's parents the option of removing guns they have in the home temporarily until Joshua's issues have resolved.

Discussing a violent event with school children is of paramount importance. NASP has published tip sheets for talking to children about violence. Specifically, the NASP recommends the following (National Association of School Psychologists 2016):

1. Reassure children that they are safe
2. Make time to talk
3. Keep your explanations developmentally appropriate
4. Review safety procedures
5. Observe children's emotional state
6. Limit television viewing of the events
7. Maintain a normal routine

In the aftermath of a serious violent event such as a school shooting, important decisions regarding the timeline for reopening of the school must be made. There are no guidelines or evidence to support these specific decisions, and administrators should handle each situation on a case-by-case basis. In some situations, such as the tragedy in Sandy Hook, the decision may be made to demolish the school and build a new one.

Long-Term (Legacy) Response

A violent event, particularly one in which there are fatalities, will continue to impact the witnesses and survivors for the rest of their lives. Planning for these years- and decades-long impacts would overwhelm even the most well-funded school districts. Simply stated, it is nearly impossible to plan in advance for the long-term responses to a violent event before the event itself has transpired. Nevertheless, the IACP has some suggestions regarding the importance of the creation of memorials and incident anniversaries. Specifically, the IACP recommends the following (International Association of Chiefs of Police and Bureau of Justice Assistance 2009):

1. Include students, families of victims, and community members in planning for memorials
2. Assess whether families want recognition of victims at graduation ceremonies, at assemblies, in yearbooks, and on anniversaries of the crisis
3. Particularly at graduations, chairs could be left empty for students who have been impacted and their names can be read

Gang Violence

Most youth-related firearm violence does not come from school mass shooters. Gang affiliation or membership increases a minor's exposure to firearm violence as well as provides a personal network for obtaining a firearm illegally (Roberto et al. 2018). Being part of a criminal street gang increases a minor's risk for both criminal offending and violent victimization (National Gang Center 2018a). Once a juvenile is exposed to firearm violence, his or her risk for subsequent gun carrying increases dramatically. In one sample of 1,170 racially/ethnically diverse male juvenile offenders, researchers found that an adolescent's odds of carrying a gun increased by more than 40% following exposure to gun violence (Beardslee et al. 2018). Understanding a student's risk for joining a gang and the possible consequences associated with gang membership can affect the individual with regard to treatment planning as well as the school and community in general.

Overview of Youth and Gangs

Gangs, often referred to as *street gangs*, *youth gangs*, or *criminal street gangs*, can be defined legally by individual state and federal statutes. In general, criteria used to define gangs include the following (National Gang Center 2018a):

- The group has three or more members who are typically ages 12–24
- Members have a shared identity linked with a name and symbols
- Members view themselves as a gang
- The group is recognized by others as a gang
- Some longevity and organization are involved
- The group has elevated involvement in criminal activity

In 2012, there were an estimated 30,700 gangs and 850,000 gang members throughout 3,100 jurisdictions in the United States, or 30% of the responding surveyed jurisdictions. In 2012, as measured by percentage of agencies reporting gang problems, gang activity was highest in larger cities (86%), followed by suburban counties (50%), smaller cities (25%), and rural counties (16%) (National Gang Center 2019). In 2016, 11% of students ages 12–18 years reported that gangs were present at school, a decline from 20% of students reporting gang presence at school in 2001. In 2016, the gang presence varied by setting, including 15% of students in urban areas, 10% in suburban areas, 4% in rural areas, 11% in public schools, and 2% in private schools (Musu-Gillette et al. 2018).

Although estimates vary, approximately 8% of youth report joining a gang by their 20s (Pyrooz 2013). Thus, the vast majority of youth do not join gangs. Some of the most common reasons why youth join gangs include increasing reputation and social status; to be with gang-involved friends or family; temptations such as money, drugs, or excitement; the culture of the gang; or identifying with their neighborhood. Some individuals join for perceived protection in a high-crime neighborhood or because of fear of the consequences of not joining (National Gang Center 2018a). Middle school age is a particularly risky time period because youth begin to spend time with other gang members and may gradually join a gang. Multiple risk factors are involved for youth who join gangs, but often, youth who are engaging in more frequent or severe delinquent behaviors are at particular risk for joining a gang (Howell 2010).

Once a youth joins a gang, the consequences can be catastrophic. Being in a gang is associated with both increased criminal offending and victimization of violent crime, a notable finding given that some youth join gangs for protection. When individuals remain in gangs for more prolonged periods of time, longer-term consequences include higher risk of dropping out of school, early parenthood, lack of stable employment, being arrested, having a criminal record, incarceration, alcohol and drug use, and poor general and mental health during adulthood (National Gang Center 2018a).

Fortunately, studies consistently find that most youth who join gangs do not remain in gangs (Howell 2007; Pyrooz 2013). In fact, the average active time youth spend in a gang is 1–2 years for the majority of youth, with less than 10% of youth spending 4 or more years involved in a gang (National Gang Center 2018a). However, youth who are more embedded in a gang or who have formed their identity as part of the gang are at greater risk for remaining in a gang for longer or are slower to desist from gangs (Pyrooz et al. 2013). Much like the process of joining a gang, leaving a gang (desistance) is also a gradual process. Some of the more common reasons individuals cite for gang desistance include growing out of the gang lifestyle, disillusionment, settling down or having family needs, and the exposure to gang violence and risk of victimization (National Gang Center 2018a).

Gang Prevention and Intervention Programs

Strategies for early intervention include intervention at the individual level with at-risk children, family prevention, and school- and community-level prevention. Prevention programs target youth at risk for gangs. Intervention programs provide services for younger youth who are already actively involved in gangs, with the intent to push them away from gangs. Law enforcement suppression targets and rehabilitates criminally active gang members who are often older and more violent. Schools and other government and community organizations may deliver services at the primary prevention level (Howell 2010). Strategies are more effective if they address risk or protective factors at the time of or before gang involvement.

Strategies are comprehensive and include communities, families, and schools to address the increased risk factors for joining a gang. Schools can be helpful by providing training for teachers on managing disruptive students; reducing suspensions and expulsions by reviewing and softening zero-tolerance policies; providing tutoring for students with poor academic performance; increasing adult supervision after school; offering interpersonal skills training for student conflict resolution; providing gang awareness training for school personnel, parents, and students; teaching students about the dangers involved in gangs; and training SROs in conflict mediation (Howell 2010).

The National Gang Center (2018b) provides a program matrix for reviewing existing gang prevention, intervention, and suppression programs as well as delinquency programs. Examples of programs that meet criteria for effective gang prevention and intervention programs for youth are included in Table 7–2.

We also want to point out the potential benefits of community-based services for preventing gang membership and helping young members navigate a path out of gangs. One such example is the Gang Rescue and Support Project (GRASP; http://graspyouth.org) based in Denver, Colorado. GRASP is a peer-led program for youth who are at risk for joining gangs, youth who are already in gangs, and their families (Hritz and Gabow 1997). There is little published on the impact of such programs at present, and this is certainly an area that is ripe for research. The National Gang Center website (www.nationalgangcenter.gov) provides guides for assessing community gang problems and implementing intervention and prevention strategies via the Office of Juvenile Justice and Delinquency Prevention's Comprehensive Gang Model.

Resources for Families

Schools can also help educate families regarding the risk that youth will join a gang, possible consequences of gang membership, and warning signs that children may be involved in a gang. The following resources are available online for free and can be provided to families readily:

- National Gang Center: Parents' Guide to Gangs, available at www.nationalgangcenter.gov/Content/Documents/Parents-Guide-to-Gangs.pdf
- American Academy of Child and Adolescent Psychiatry: Gangs and Children, available at www.aacap.org/AACAP/Families_and_Youth/Facts_for_Families/FFF-Guide/Children-and-Gangs-098.aspx
- American Academy of Pediatrics (HealthyChildren.org): Teenagers and Gangs, available at www.healthychildren.org/English/ages-stages/teen/Pages/Teenagers-and-Gangs.aspx

TABLE 7–2. **Examples of effective gang prevention and intervention programs for youth**

Program	Description
Broader Urban Involvement and Leadership Development (BUILD) Violence Intervention Curriculum	Prevention program to help youth (ages 13–14) in detention by providing counseling, community education, and work-readiness training through a prevention program, intervention program, community resource development program, and rehabilitation program
Caught in the Crossfire (Oakland, California)	Comprehensive program targeting individuals (ages 12–25) who have been admitted to the hospital with a violence-related injury to provide intervention for coping and considering alternatives to retaliation
Chicago Alternative Policing Strategy (CAPS)	Intervention program targeting individuals ages 10–24 that includes a community-based policing strategy in which officers work with neighborhood residents to identify crime problems and determine solutions
Gang Resistance Education and Training (GREAT)	Prevention program for youth ages 8–14 that includes a 13-week course taught in the classroom by uniformed law enforcement officers to reduce risk factors and increase protective factors
Group Violence Intervention (GVI)	Suppression program targeting individuals ages 15–21 to engage those actively involved in violent street gangs to reduce violence and homicide
Hardcore Gang Investigations Unit—Los Angeles County District Attorney's Office	Suppression program for individuals ages 12–30 that involves targeting and prosecuting the most violent and habitual gang offenders through vertical prosecution
San Diego County Breaking Cycles	Intervention program for youth ages 12–17 that includes prevention for youth who have not yet entered the juvenile justice system but exhibit problematic behaviors and graduated sanctions for those in juvenile court for delinquency involvement

Key Points

- Mass school shootings are rare events, whereas other forms of violent and nonviolent victimization at school are more common.
- The options-based approach to dealing with armed school intruders is otherwise known as "run, hide, and fight."
- Most youth who join gangs eventually leave the gang lifestyle.

Clinical Pearls

There is no reliable profile of school shooters.

The use of metal detectors to mitigate violent acts at school lacks empirical support.

The presence of guns in the home increases the likelihood of both suicide and homicide among household members.

References

Advanced Law Enforcement Rapid Response Training Center, Federal Bureau of Investigation: Active Shooter Incidents in the United States in 2016 and 2017. Washington, DC, Federal Bureau of Investigation, U.S. Department of Justice, 2018

Allely CS, Wilson P, Minnis H, et al: Violence is rare in autism: when it does occur, is it sometimes extreme? J Psychol 151(1):49–68, 2017 27185105

Ash P: School shootings and mental illness, in Gun Violence and Mental Illness. Edited by Gold LH, Simon RI. Arlington, VA, American Psychiatric Association Publishing, 2016, pp 105–126

Beardslee J, Mulvey E, Schubert C, et al: Gun- and non-gun-related violence exposure and risk for subsequent gun carrying among male juvenile offenders. J Am Acad Child Adolesc Psychiatry 57(4):274–279, 2018 29588053

Centers for Disease Control and Prevention: Youth Violence: Using Environmental Design to Prevent School Violence. Atlanta, GA, Centers for Disease Control and Prevention, 2018. Available at: www.cdc.gov/violenceprevention/youthviolence/cpted.html. Accessed August 9, 2018.

Diliberti M, Jackson M, Kemp J: Crime, Violence, Discipline, and Safety in U.S. Public Schools: Findings From the School Survey on Crime and Safety: 2015–16 (NCES 2017-122). Washington, DC, U.S. National Center for Education Statistics, Department of Education, 2017. Available at: https://nces.ed.gov/pubs2017/2017122.pdf. Accessed August 9, 2018.

Fox JA, Fridel EE: The tenuous connections involving mass shootings, mental illness, and gun laws. Violence Gend 3(1):14–19, 2016

Frattaroli S, McGinty EE, Barnhorst A, et al: Gun violence restraining orders: alternative or adjunct to mental health-based restrictions on firearms? Behav Sci Law 33(2–3):290–307, 2015 25990840

Giffords Law Center to Prevent Gun Violence: Gun Laws by Policy Area. San Francisco, CA, Giffords Law Center to Prevent Gun Violence, 2018. Available at: https://lawcenter.giffords.org/search-gun-law-by-gun-policy. Accessed October 11, 2018.

Gun Control Act of 1968, § 101, Pub. L. No. 90-618, 82 Stat. 123

Hankin A, Hertz M, Simon T: Impacts of metal detector use in schools: insights from 15 years of research. J Sch Health 81(2):100–106, 2011 21223277

Howell JC: Menacing or mimicking? Realities of youth gangs. Juv Fam Court J 58(2):39–50, 2007

Howell JC: Gang Prevention: An Overview of Research and Programs. Juvenile Justice Bulletin. Washington, DC, Office of Juvenile Justice and Delinquency Prevention, December 2010

Hritz SA, Gabow PA: A peer approach to high risk youth. J Adolesc Health 20(4):259–260, 1997 9098728

International Association of Chiefs of Police, Bureau of Justice Assistance: Guide for Preventing and Responding to School Violence, 2nd Edition. Alexandria, VA, International Association of Chiefs of Police, 2009. Available at: www.bja.gov/Publications/IACP_School_Violence.pdf. Accessed March 26, 2019.

Jones RT, Randall J: Rehearsal-plus: Coping with fire emergencies and reducing fire-related fears. Fire Technology 4:432–444, 1994

Kellermann AL, Rivara FP, Somes G, et al: Suicide in the home in relation to gun ownership. N Engl J Med 327(7):467–472, 1992 1308093

Kellermann AL, Rivara FP, Rushforth NB, et al: Gun ownership as a risk factor for homicide in the home. N Engl J Med 329(15):1084–1091, 1993 8371731

Knoll JL 4th: The "pseudocommando" mass murderer: part I, the psychology of revenge and obliteration. J Am Acad Psychiatry Law, 38(1):87–94, 2010a 20305080

Knoll JL 4th: The "pseudocommando" mass murderer: part II, the language of revenge. J Am Acad Psychiatry Law 38(2):263–272, 2010b 20542949

Miltenberger RG, Gatheridge BJ, Satterlund M, et al: Teaching safety skills to children to prevent gun play: an evaluation of in situ training. J Appl Behav Anal 38(3):395–398, 2005 16270848

Musu-Gillette L, Zhang A, Wang K, et al: Indicators of School Crime and Safety: 2017 (NCES 2018-036/NCJ 251413). Washington, DC, National Center for Education Statistics, U.S. Department of Education, 2018

National Association of School Psychologists: Talking to Children About Violence: Tips for Parents and Teachers. Bethesda, MD, National Association of School Psychologists, 2016. Available at: www.nasponline.org/resources-and-publications/resources/school-safety-and-crisis/talking-to-children-about-violence-tips-for-parents-and-teachers. Accessed August 9, 2018.

National Association of School Psychologists, National Association of School Resource Officers: Best Practice Considerations for Schools in Active Shooter and Other Armed Assailant Drills. Bethesda, MD, National Association of School Psychologists, 2014

National Association of School Psychologists, National Association of School Resource Officers: Best Practice Considerations for Schools in Active Shooter and Other Armed Assailant Drills. (Updated) Bethesda, MD, National Association of School Psychologists, 2017

National Association of School Resource Officers: About NASRO. Hoover, AL, National Association of School Resource Officers, 2018. Available at: https://nasro.org/about. Accessed August 9, 2018.

National Gang Center: Frequently asked questions about gangs. Washington, DC, National Gang Center, 2018a. Available at www.nationalgangcenter.gov/About/FAQ. Accessed October 6, 2018.

National Gang Center: Strategic Planning Tool: Program Matrix. Washington, DC, National Gang Center, 2018b. Available at: www.nationalgangcenter.gov/SPT/Program-Matrix. Accessed October 7, 2018.

National Gang Center: National Youth Gang Survey Analysis. Washington, DC, National Gang Center, 2019. Available at: www.nationalgangcenter.gov/Survey-Analysis. Accessed March 30, 2019.

Neuman Y, Assaf D, Cohen Y, et al: Profiling school shooters: automatic text-based analysis. Front Psychiatry 6:86, 2015 26089804

O'Toole ME: The School Shooter: A Threat Assessment Perspective. Quantico, VA, National Center for the Analysis of Violent Crime, Federal Bureau of Investigation, 2000

Pyrooz DC: "From your first cigarette to your last dyin' day": the patterning of gang membership in the life-course. J Quant Criminol 30(2):349–372, 2013

Pyrooz DC, Sweeten G, Piquero AR: Continuity and change in gang membership and gang embeddedness. Journal of Research in Crime and Delinquency 50(2):239–271, 2013

Roberto E, Braga AA, Papachristos AV: Closer to guns: the role of street gangs in facilitating access to illegal firearms. J Urban Health 95(3):372–382, 2018 29744717

Rose S, Bisson J, Churchill R, et al: Psychological debriefing for preventing post traumatic stress disorder (PTSD). Cochrane Database Syst Rev (2):CD000560, 2002 12076399

Schaechter J, Alvarez PG: Growing up—or not—with gun violence. Pediatr Clin North Am 63(5):813–826, 2016 27565360

Stone MH: Mass murder, mental Illness, and men. Violence Gend 2(1):51–88, 2015

Vossekuil B, Fein R, Reddy M, et al: The Final Report and Findings of the Safe School Initiative: Implications for the Prevention of School Attacks in the United States. Washington, DC, Safe and Drug-Free Schools Program, Office of Elementary and Secondary Education, U.S. Department of Education, 2002

Zhe EJ, Nickerson AB: Effects of an intruder crisis drill on children's knowledge, anxiety, and perceptions of school safety. School Psych Rev 36(3):501–508, 2007

PART II
Threat and Risk Assessment

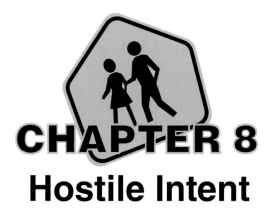

CHAPTER 8
Hostile Intent

The Principles of Threat Assessment

Michael B. Kelly, M.D.

Anne B. McBride, M.D.

Jeff Bostic, M.D., Ed.D.

Sharon Hoover, Ph.D.

Arany Uthayakumar, B.A.

…[N]ever neglect an extraordinary appearance or happening. It may be—usually is, in fact—a false alarm that leads to nothing, but may on the other hand be the clue provided by fate to lead you to some important advance.

Sir Alexander Fleming

Case Vignette

Justin is a 15-year-old boy referred by his regular therapist for mental health crisis evaluation. During one of his weekly therapy sessions, he informed his therapist that he planned to blow up his high school. Given his mental health history and the possibility of imminent danger to others, Justin's therapist was concerned he might meet criteria for psychiatric hospitalization.

On crisis evaluation, Justin reports that he plans to "blow up the school." When asked about further steps he has taken to achieve this plan, he states that he currently does not have any explosives or materials to build explosives but has been doing online research on how to build explosives. When asked about his motive for blowing up the school, he reports that he feels angry at the school and students who attend the school. He notes that he is no longer attending his high school because he had transitioned to an independent studies program following a decline in his grades earlier in the school year.

Justin reports that he also plans to kill his mother's boyfriend. He states that the boyfriend is "a worthless piece of trash" and that he is "100% sure" he would kill the boyfriend if he had a gun. When asked about his access to firearms and other weapons, Justin provides a vague response. He notes that his mother's boyfriend has been staying with him and his mother too often and has complained to Justin about his behavior, which Justin asserts is "none of his business."

It can be helpful to distinguish *threat* from *risk* when evaluating a person's risk for harming others. A *threat* is a specific statement or action that communicates intent to harm people or property, also known as *targeted violence.* Threats serve a variety of purposes. In some cases, threats serve the purpose of intimidating a person or group of people. In other situations, threats may convey the intent to do physical harm. Threats can be characterized in a manner similar to how we define aggression and its subtypes in Chapter 2, "A Recipe for Violence." That is, a threat may underlie a highly calculated plan to harm a specific person or group or may represent an unfiltered comment from an upset person who is unlikely to carry out threatened violence after calming down.

Evaluating the credibility and seriousness of a threat (i.e., performing a threat assessment) generally requires a team approach toward clarifying the intentions and capabilities of the threatening party (O'Toole 2000). The main objectives of a threat assessment are to gather as much information as possible about a threat, determine its seriousness (does the threat represent a transient or impulsive statement, or is it a substantive plan to cause harm created by persons with the means to carry it out?), develop a strategy to protect potential victims, and, if possible, eliminate or mitigate problems that give rise to the threat.

Risk refers to a person's ongoing capacity and intention to act on a threat. Violence risk refers to factors that make a person more or less likely to engage in violent behavior. In other words, a person may not intend to immediately follow through on a particular threat or may quickly change his or her mind. However, the factors that gave rise to the threat in the first place or that cause potential victims to be vulnerable to harm may remain. For example, even threats that are reactive, impulsive, and of time-limited duration can be acted on in the heat of the moment or at a later time if the circumstances that triggered the threat return. A violence risk assessment is thus a dynamic process that seeks to characterize the likelihood of a person hurting others along a continuum from low to moderate to high. Determinations of risk are based on identifiable risk factors (static and dynamic) and protective factors. The ultimate goal of a risk assessment is to create a plan that addresses a student's treatment needs and protects potential victims from harm. We provide a more detailed review of violence risk assessment in Chapter 9, "Avoiding Danger."

Overview of Threat Assessment

Following the 1999 Columbine school shootings, both the Federal Bureau of Investigation (FBI) and the United States Secret Service in collaboration with the U.S. Department of Education developed reports on targeted school violence. Neither group concluded that a profile for the typical school shooter existed, and both groups argued for the use of a threat assessment model to prevent possible future school violence. As the FBI report noted, "All threats are NOT created equal" (O'Toole 2000). The report emphasized that rather than zero-tolerance policies against school violence, schools should implement a threat assessment approach to analyze the credibility and seriousness of the threat as well as the extent of the resources, intent, and motivation the student possesses to carry out the threat. The authors of the report advocated for use of a four-pronged model for threat assessments that includes the following four major areas: personality of the student, family dynamics, school dynamics and the student's role in those dynamics, and social dynamics.

Findings from the Safe School Initiative, conducted by the Secret Service and the Department of Education, were based on the review of 37 incidents of targeted school violence and included some common features (Vossekuil et al. 2002). Notably, most incidents of targeted violence were planned, other people had advance knowledge of the attacker's ideas or plans, and most of the attackers were behaving in ways that caused prior concern from other people. Such commonalities indicated that some future attacks may be preventable, and therefore, use of a threat assessment approach may be a helpful strategy for preventing school-based attacks (Vossekuil et al. 2002).

The Virginia Model for Student Threat Assessment (Cornell and Sheras 2006, updated by Cornell 2018) was developed in response to the FBI and Secret Service reports as guidelines to be used by school administrators in response to threat of violence by a student. Once a threat is reported, the Virginia Model follows five possible steps. The first step involves evaluating the threat, which includes interviewing the student who made the threat, as well as witnesses, to determine the threat context and clarifying what the threat was meant to convey and the associated intentions. The second step is to decide whether the threat is clearly transient or substantive. According to the FBI (O'Toole 2000), indicators of substantive threats may include the following:

1. The threat includes plausible details (e.g., persons involved, time, place, methods)
2. The threat has been discussed with multiple people over an identifiable period of time
3. The threat was described as a plan, or there is evidence that planning has begun
4. The student has involved peers or attempted to recruit peers in the planning process
5. A proclamation has been made to peers who are invited to witness the threat being put into action
6. There is physical evidence that is consistent with the student's threat (e.g., knife, firearm, instructions for making explosives)

If the threat is deemed transient, the next step is to respond to the transient threat. If the threat is substantive, the team responds with further measures, including protective action. The team determines whether the substantive threat is serious (threat to assault, strike, or beat up someone) or very serious (threat to kill, sexually assault, or severely injure someone). The model advocates for responding to all substantive threats. If the threat is determined to be very serious, in steps 4 and 5, a safety evaluation is conducted and a safety plan is implemented.

The Virginia Model recommends that each school have a threat assessment team that includes an administrator, a law enforcement representative, and one or more mental health professionals. In the most serious cases, the school psychologist or mental health professional conducts a mental health evaluation, following a risk reduction or risk management approach. Field tests have shown promising support for this model (Cornell 2011).

Threat Assessment Process

Increasingly, school administrators, sometimes with assistance from school mental health clinicians, will attempt to discern whether a threat made by a student is transient or substantive. Of note, approximately 70% of threats made at school are transient (Cornell et al. 2004). If the threat is transient and if there is no evidence or pattern of worsening student functioning, then the threat may be addressed within the school's policies. However, sometimes, the school administrators turn over the evaluation to others (e.g., law enforcement, mental health professionals outside of school) who may seek information from a variety of persons with knowledge about the context of the threat (e.g., other school staff, parents, peers, the individual(s) being targeted). A structured approach to threat assessment, such as implementation of the Virginia Student Threat Assessment Guidelines, is a useful method for systematically addressing targeted violence.

Threat Assessment Team

As described by Cornell and Sheras (2006), each individual school benefits from forming its own threat assessment team. Staff within the school will be most familiar with how their students, including the potential perpetrator(s) and target(s), interact, the circumstances surrounding the threat, and the school's culture and how these factors might influence expression of a threat. In addition, a school-based team diminishes the disruption to the school from an outside team appearing to conduct a threat assessment. Outside teams take longer to form and to reach the school, and their input, if not attuned to what is feasible for the school, can be problematic. Ultimately, the task of altering factors contributing to a given threat will be handled by the school, so it stands to reason that the school's investment in the threat assessment process will be greater if it plays a significant role throughout. In general, it is preferable for multiple school team members to be involved in the threat assessment; the decisions made about the student; disciplinary procedures, if any; and interactions with law enforcement, if needed. Schools vary in their resources and staffing, so some roles may or may not be feasible at a particular school.

School Team Members

Staffing at schools is widely diverse, so team configurations will necessarily vary. A school administrator (e.g., principal, assistant principal) is vital because that person functions in the roles of making the school effective, supporting each student, and considering the impact of any intervention on all the other students in the building. The administrator has the authority to make decisions in the best interest of everyone in the school and can usually manage most threats expeditiously.

School mental health clinicians (e.g., psychologists, school counselors, school social workers) are particularly helpful because of the following: 1) their familiarity with child development and mental health is helpful in identifying psychopathology (e.g., trauma, anxiety, depression, delusions) that might underlie threats or related events, and 2) they often know the provoking factors, where the perpetrator "fits" within the school population, and available interventions in the school or community that may alter the student's level of threat. In sum, the school mental health clinician's role on the threat assessment team involves helping to contextualize precipitating events, motives, and other factors. The role of mental health clinicians in a risk assessment model includes helping to alter the variables giving rise to threats. This is elaborated on in Chapter 9.

Law Enforcement Team Members

Law enforcement officers are a vital part of the threat assessment team. In the event of serious threats or risks to others, law enforcement officers are best trained and prepared to provide protection. In addition, when laws are broken (e.g., threats, assaults, weapons brought to school), students may become entwined with the juvenile justice system. Thus, law enforcement officers who are familiar with the local juvenile justice system are an invaluable resource. Furthermore, law enforcement officers are the most qualified members of the team to execute on-campus searches for evidence (e.g., weapons, drugs) when necessary. Ideally, school resource officers (SROs), if available in a school, are preferred because they know the particular school's culture and may have familiarity and/or rapport with the students involved. In fact, a 2005 report submitted to the U.S. Department of Justice (Finn and McDevitt 2005) showed that one of the biggest factors in the successful use of SROs is creating a rapport with the student body such that the SRO is trusted and regarded positively.

There is a growing body of literature suggesting that SROs are helpful in a number of ways, such as by reducing the incidents of arrest on campus. They may also increase the level of comfort students have with reporting threats made by other members of the student body (Finn 2006; Finn and McDevitt 2005; Theriot 2009). However, SROs are less helpful when their role is perceived as being that of an enforcer for school administration (Ryan et al. 2017). Furthermore, perceptions of school safety can vary depending on students' ethnic background and history of victimization. For instance, a recent study by Theriot and Orme (2016) surveyed nearly 2,000 middle and high school students and found that African American students as well as those with a history of past victimization felt less safe regardless of their level of interaction with SROs. In general, male students, those with positive attitudes toward SROs, and students who were more connected with the school and peers reported feeling the safest. These data underscore the complex relationship that schools, students, and their communities have with law enforcement while also highlighting that more research is needed in this area.

Teachers

Teachers are rarely part of the threat assessment team because they do not have the authority to make decisions or have specialized training in gauging and evaluating threats. However, in some schools, teachers may serve various functions when needed. For example, schools that do not have mental health clinicians may rely on a special education teacher who, within that school, may have the most training and awareness with regard to mental health.

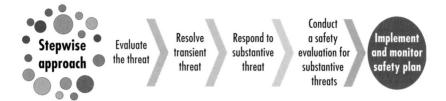

FIGURE 8–1. **Five steps of the Virginia Model for Student Threat Assessment guidelines.**
Adapted from Cornell 2018.

Stepwise Approach to Threat Assessment

When a threat is made, rapid response is necessary. The threat assessment team is assembled, and the school administrator and/or threat assessment team evaluates the threat. Usually, the administrator will separately interview the alleged perpetrator, target, and peers or staff who may have useful knowledge (e.g., close friends of the alleged perpetrator or target, parents, coaches) or were present when the threat was made. On the basis of the recommendations of the seminal work by Cornell and Sheras (2006), *Guidelines for Responding to Student Threats of Violence,* we recommend that school administrators follow a systematic and stepwise approach to assessing threats (Figure 8–1). The following steps incorporate an updated overview (Cornell 2018), with the caveat that we wish to emphasize the importance of having some degree of safety assessment and creating a safety plan in regard to all substantive threats.

Step 1: Evaluate the Threat

It is important for school personnel to write down exactly what they have heard or seen from those involved regarding the threat. Obtaining an accurate record of what is said or done is critical for both evaluating the threat and ensuring transparency throughout the process. In addition, it is paramount to determine, as much as possible, what was happening around the time the threat was made and whether the threat was in response to an identifiable precipitating event. The threatening student is typically interviewed during this first step.

Step 2: Attempt to Resolve Transient Threat

The credibility and seriousness of the threat is evaluated in step 2. After identifying a potential threat, the next step involves determining whether the threat is transient (i.e., short lived and quick to resolve) versus substantive (i.e., a threat in which the desire to harm someone endures) in nature. Transient threats, much like our description of "hot" aggression in Chapter 2, are often made in the heat of the moment in response to an identifiable trigger. For example, a student who threatens to injure a peer in response to being ridiculed will likely calm down once the parties are given an opportunity to simmer down and possibly resolve their differences. However, a chronically ridiculed student who tells a friend about well-formulated plans to harm the offending party when he or she least suspects it is making a substantive threat. Not all threats can be accounted for in an either/or fashion, so it is recommended that school administrators err on the side of caution and regard threats as substantive in the face of uncertainty. See Table 8–1 for a brief description of different types of threats with associated examples.

A threat that is identified as transient in nature can be addressed however the school normally handles such incidents (e.g., calling parents, fostering discussion between feuding students, taking disciplinary action). Of note, even transient threats that resolve quickly can be associated with psychopathology that warrants formal intervention and, in some cases, safety planning. For example, a transient threat made in the context of ongoing depression or untreated posttraumatic stress disorder will warrant more than a brief conflict resolution exercise and may be the student's first point of contact for much-needed mental health services.

Step 3: Respond to a Substantive Threat

All substantive threats must be responded to quickly and comprehensively and require protective action (e.g., notifying the intended victim and his or her parents or guardians as well as the parents or guardians of the student who made the threat, increased supervision of students involved). Cornell and Sheras (2006) recommended differentiating between threats that are *serious* (e.g., threatening to beat up a peer) versus those that are *very serious* (e.g., threatening to sexually assault or kill a peer). In our view, there can be much overlap between threats that are considered serious and those that are very serious. In responding to a substantive threat, the team should also look for ways to resolve the conflict and provide appropriate discipline when necessary.

Step 4: Conduct a Safety Evaluation for Substantive Threats

Cornell and Sheras (2006) recommended a formal safety evaluation for all very serious threats. As updated (Cornell 2018), the model includes protective actions as in step 3, screening for mental health services or providing counseling, law enforcement investigation of the case, and integrating findings from the mental health and law enforcement evaluations into a safety plan.

We additionally contend that all substantive threats require some degree of safety assessment because the severity of the threat does not

TABLE 8–1. **Types of threats**

Type	Description	Example
Transient	Short lived and quick to resolve	"I wanted to punch Jimmy when he cut me in line, and I almost did it, too."
Substantive	Characterized by an enduring desire to harm another person	"I don't care if Ross apologized; this is not over. I'm gonna get him after school."
Direct	Plainly identifies a specific target	"We are gonna jump Tina by the library after sixth period."
Indirect	Concerning statements that are ambiguous or vague	"Jorge and his homies think I'm soft. They'll find out I'm not soon enough."
Veiled	Implies pending violence without stating explicitly	"Miriam, you need to be careful nothing happens to you walking through that neighborhood after school. You never know what might happen."
Conditional	Threat used as leverage to achieve a desired outcome	"If you don't pay me the $100 you owe, plus another $50, we're gonna beat your ass."

Source.   Adapted from Cornell and Sheras 2006; O'Toole 2000.

necessarily correlate with an individual's risk and needs. In fact, in psychiatry in general, safety planning is often involved in clinical encounters. Although we agree with the information from Cornell and Sheras' (2006) decision tree, we wish to emphasize that, at a bare minimum, some degree of safety assessment is warranted for all substantive threats. For example, although not all threats to assault a peer will warrant law enforcement involvement, the student may still benefit from a screen for mental health services and referral to appropriate resources.

Thus, in general, we recommend responding to substantive threats by 1) taking immediate steps to protect intended victims and notifying their parents, 2) notifying the parents of the student who has made the substantive threat, 3) beginning a mental health evaluation of the student and referring him or her for clinical services and other interventions as appropriate, 4) considering contacting law enforcement for serious threats and consulting with law enforcement in cases of very serious threats (i.e., those with the potential for loss of life, sexual assault, or other extreme injuries), and 5) disciplining the student as appropriate.

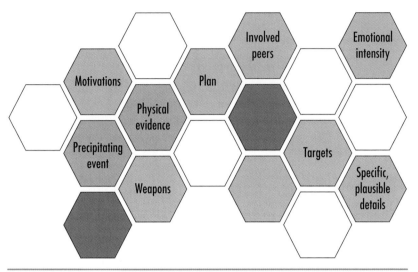

FIGURE 8–2. **Mosaic of interacting factors analyzed during threat assessment.**

Step 5: Implement and Monitor the Safety Plan

We recommend creating a safety plan for students in response to both serious and very serious threats. The extent of the safety plan can vary a great deal depending on the types of threats made and risk factors for serious violence, which we elaborate on in Chapter 5, "Bullying and Cyberbullying." As Cornell and Sheras (2006) indicated, the safety plan should be documented in a written format and be subject to revision when appropriate, and contact should be maintained with the student.

Threat Assessment Content

In some cases, a threat assessment may be completed and terminated within an hour. For example, situations where a perceived threat has a low potential for harm, low intention, and little probability of being acted on will not require extensive evaluation. In contrast, with situations in which the student making the threat feels justified in doing so, has a specified plan in mind, and harbors multiple violence risk factors in the setting of an ongoing conflict, a more extensive approach is indicated. Thus, the content of threat assessments will vary on the basis of the types of threats and the contexts in which they occur. Factors relevant to threat assessment are shown in Figure 8–2, and Table 8–2 includes some examples of questions that may be helpful when performing a threat assessment, based largely on O'Toole's (2000) FBI report on school shooters.

TABLE 8–2. Components of a threat assessment and sample questions

Component	Description	Sample questions
Precipitating event	Event(s) surrounding a specific threat	What led up to this threat? Did anything happen that pushed the student over the edge to make this threat? What was going on when this threat was made?
Physical evidence	Actual evidence relevant to the threat (e.g., e-mails, text messages, weapons); most commonly found in backpack, locker, or bedroom or on cell phone or other devices	Did the student write anything to anyone about this threat? Did anyone receive any texts, letters, or e-mails about this threat? Did the student have any weapons on him or her at school to enact the threat?
Motivations	Potential motives of the student in making a threat	What reasons did the student and others give for making this threat? What did the student anticipate would happen after making this threat (e.g., causing others to retreat, intimidation)?
Plan	Plan (if any) surrounding execution of the threat	Did the student (or anyone else) make plans for enacting the threat? How sophisticated was the plan? Had the student who made the threat taken steps to prepare or follow through with this plan?
Involved peers	Peers with whom the student may have communicated or planned in making a threat	Did the student talk to other students or adults about this threat or target(s)? Was anyone encouraging the student making the threat to make or enact a threat?

TABLE 8–2.   **Components of a threat assessment and sample questions** *(continued)*

Component	Description	Sample questions
Targets	Identity of alleged person(s) being targeted and the reason for being targeted	How did the person become the target? Was the threat made in the setting of an ongoing conflict or because of someone having a bad day (e.g., wrong place at the wrong time)? What about the target(s) and/or situation caused the student to go forward with making threats?
Weapons	Any weapons that may have been associated with a threat	Did the threat involve any mention of weapons? Does the student who made the threat have access to weapons? Has the student who made the threat used weapons in the past?
Specific, plausible details	Specific details related to the threat (e.g., "stab you with my uncle's knife" vs. "you should be blown up") and their plausibility (e.g., "I have my uncle's knife at home" vs. the student having no clue how to make a bomb)	How did the student who made the threat describe harming the target(s)? How specific were details of this plan? Had the student making the threat completed various steps of the plan (e.g., obtained weapons, identified a place and time to act)? How plausible are the student's threat and associated plan, if any?
Emotional intensity	Threats made in the heat of the moment (RADI aggression) versus threats that are cold and calculated in nature (PIP aggression)	What was the student's apparent emotional state at the time of the threat (e.g., cold and detached vs. hot and lashing out)? Does the student who made the threat recall his or her emotional state (e.g., "I was really pissed off!") around the time of the incident? Is the self-reported emotional state of the student who made the threat similar to the perception of witnesses (e.g., peers, teachers)?

Abbreviations.   PIP=planned, instrumental, and predatory; RADI=reactive, affective, defensive, and impulsive.

Precipitating Events

The immediate events surrounding a threat should be clarified. Specifically, seemingly unrelated events, such as conflicts with family or receiving bad news about unrelated topics, may be displaced onto others or the school. Precipitating events that directly involve the target(s) or are emblematic of ongoing frustrations, particularly at school, are more concerning.

Physical Evidence

Types of physical evidence that convey a plan to act on a threat or have the potential to cause great harm are most concerning (e.g., notes, e-mails, or text messages outlining a plan; attempts to obtain weapons). Such evidence is often found in the student's backpack, locker, car, or bedroom or on personal electronic devices (Tom 2014). Finding physical evidence can be difficult because parents may be needed to find such evidence at home. Similarly, schools must be mindful of legal search and seizure parameters, so law enforcement engagement may be necessary to clarify options for searching a potential or alleged perpetrator's personal property (e.g., backpack, locker, car) both inside and outside school.

Motivations

Most often, children and adolescents make threats in response to anger or frustration with little forethought and a low likelihood of acting on them. For instance, younger children may make threats in retaliation or in an attempt to get what they want ("If you don't let me eat ice cream now, I'll kick you"). Middle school students may make threats in defense of peers ("If they suspend you, I'll tear up the classroom"). High school and college students may make threats related to strongly held personal beliefs (e.g., "If they don't allow us to protest [a political candidate's appearance], we'll torch the student center"). Multiple motivations may underlie the threat, including retaliation, extortion, or intimidation, so exploring possible motivations is important.

Prior Communication of Threats

Students often communicate their thoughts, fantasies, or plans to hurt others in advance. This process is referred to as *leakage* (O'Toole 2000) and can serve as both a warning and a cry for help (Table 8–3). Students are often the best eyes and ears to pick up leakage and should be educated on their potential role in keeping the campus safe by looking out for each other rather than thinking of it as snitching.

TABLE 8–3.   **Advance communication of threats**

Leakage

  May be intentional or unintentional

  Offers clues to feelings, thoughts, fantasies, attitudes, or intentions that may
    signal an impending violent act

  Includes subtle threats, boasts, innuendos, predictions, or ultimatums

  May be spoken or conveyed in stories, diary entries, essays, poems, letters,
    songs, drawings, doodles, tattoos, or videos

Source.   O'Toole 2000.

Targets

Identified targets, particularly the same target(s) over time, warrant
more concern than a student lashing out at different students or at the
most proximate student. Certainly, school shootings have rarely focused on one or two specific targets, operating mostly on availability
(i.e., targeting victims who are simply present rather than specifically
sought by the perpetrator). However, ongoing perceptions of mistreatment by specific others, such as peers or students, represent greater pre-
occupation and sustained focus on harming people.

Weapons

Access to and familiarity with weapons, especially firearms, increase
the seriousness of a threat. It is worth mentioning that the United States
has more gun-related fatalities for youth than all other Westernized
countries combined, although only a small percentage of fatal shootings
(0.3%) spills over into schools (Nekvasil et al. 2015).

Plan

Threats that involve more effort and multiple steps in preparation represent more danger. Similarly, plans that have been discussed with others,
particularly repetitively or recurrently, with revisions along the way, warrant greater concern than impromptu aggressive acts or threatening
statements made by students.

Specific, Plausible Details

The details surrounding a threat are pertinent. Evaluators can attempt to
discern the sincerity and plausibility of a threat by clarifying the specific
targeted individuals, the reasons given to "justify" the threat, and information on how and when the threat is to be acted, as well as whether or
not the individual has acted on previous threats. Improbable threats
("I'm going to mount a machine gun on a tank and shoot and run people
over") may be highly detailed but highly unrealistic, and they represent

something different from plausible threats. Specifically, improbable threats may represent more a person's desire to call significant attention to an interpersonal conflict than an actual desire to harm someone. This may be particularly true for younger students. Elementary and middle school students may be prone to making sincere yet implausible threats due to fear of peer rejection or retaliation if they back down in a conflict. In such cases, outlandish threats may be the only way the student believes that he or she can save face during a conflict.

Emotional Intensity and Types of Aggression

Threats characterized by emotional, reactive, and defensive displays, even when described in vivid terms ("I hate your guts—I'm going to chop you up into tiny pieces"), have not been correlated with being acted on (O'Toole 2000). Intense threats characterized by reactive, affective, defensive, and impulsive (RADI) aggression most often reflect a student's anger in that moment rather than a cold or carefully calculated plan to harm others. However, repetitive distressing, intense threats or comments over time, as have occurred with students who have kept records (e.g., journals, notes, videos) chronicling ongoing intense hostility toward others, represent a greater concern.

Collateral Reports

Threat assessment generally is most reliable when it involves multiple sources of information that can be used to understand the context, the precipitating and potentially perpetuating factors related to specific threats, and any associated risk of violence. Interviews of peers and school staff present when a threat was made, as well as the targeted student(s), should focus on identifying the potential or alleged perpetrator's motivations, intent, and likelihood of carrying out violence.

Cornell and Sheras (2006) recommended the following questions for witnesses, which require some adaptations on the basis of witnesses' ages and/or developmental levels:

1. *What exactly happened during [the incident]?* The actual events, even among people who were present, may be reported differently; therefore, conducting separate interviews with each witness is preferred and may allow greater precision.
2. *What exactly did [the perpetrator] say or do?* Obtaining the actual words or actions that composed the threat is preferable, and the sooner after the incident, usually the better.
3. *What do you think the student meant while making the alleged threat?* Getting clarity on whether the threat appeared to be a joke versus a very serious threat requires taking into account not only the words spoken but also the volume of voice and nonverbal communications (e.g., waving arms, gritting teeth, raising a fist).

4. *How did you feel about what was said or done?* Did the threat make (and leave) witnesses frightened, afraid, or distressed, or did it appear to be more like banter between people that was not of a serious nature?
5. *Do you think the student might really follow through on the threat? Are you concerned that anything else might happen?* Were there other comments or signals from the perpetrator that suggested this was more serious? In addition, did the target or others react in such a way that additional conflict may be expected? For example, if a male perpetrator threatened a female target, did anything occur to suggest that the target's boyfriend might retaliate against the perpetrator now?
6. *Do you know why the student made the threat?* Was this an unexpected escalation or a brewing problem that remains volatile? Is some further resolution needed?

Levels of Risk Surrounding a Threat

Schools will sometimes require an evaluation to determine whether a student is "safe" or "unsafe" to return to school; however, this sort of dichotomy is not consistent with modern approaches to threat and risk assessment. Threats fall on a continuum, as does the level of associated risk of violence. Table 8–4 shows how these variables help discern the level of risk of a given threat.

Evaluators can and should provide their professional opinion regarding a student's level of violence risk rather than describe a student as safe or unsafe to return to school. Evaluators cannot reliably dichotomize decisions about safety because important variables can shift over time, thereby increasing or reducing the likelihood that a specific threat will be acted on. Threats, like levels of violence risk, are dynamic, not static. The seriousness of threats is influenced by the context in which they arise and how associated variables change over time.

Threat Assessment and Confidentiality

Mental health evaluators performing formal threat assessments should inform interviewees of the nonconfidential nature of their discussion and describe the circumstances under which the information discussed will be shared (e.g., report, team meeting). Informed consent should be obtained from parents before interviewing students who are minors.

School Mental Health Provider's Duty to Protect

When school-based mental health treatment providers become aware of a serious threat of harm, their duty to protect others supersedes their duty

TABLE 8–4. Level of risk for a threat

Component	Low level of risk	Medium level of risk	High level of risk
Precipitants	Recent one-time event	Ongoing precipitant	Multiple persisting precipitants having greater impact on violence risk
Physical evidence	No or minimal evidence	Notes, texts, and/or e-mails usually limited to this event	History of notes, texts, and/or e-mails; materials to harm others pursued or obtained
Motives	Unrelated to threat or target	Related to target	Multiple or overlapping motivations related to target(s)
Plans	Poorly planned	Rough plans with holes or gaps	Persisting plan with some evidence of effort to obtain necessary means (e.g., weaponry)
Involved peers	None	Others accessed	Others participating to assist with threat or encourage increased aggression
Targets	Not identified	Specific targets may change or be different	Specific targets sustained over time
Weaponry	Low access; unfamiliar with using weapons	Access to weaponry but no history of misusing	Interest in or preoccupation with weaponry; harm to others with weapons (distinguish appropriate hunting from efforts to make animals or others suffer)
Threat details	Nonspecific, ambiguous	Specific but may be circumscribed to that moment	Details become increasingly specific, fixed, or revised and complete
Plausibility	Not realistic	Possible but improbable	Doable currently
Emotional intensity	Low or brief (minutes) emotion	May be emotional about this incident now, but targets change	Emotional about target or factors sustaining over weeks or cold and calculated threat

to maintain confidentiality. The most famous example of mental health providers' duty to protect comes from the case of Tarasoff v. Regents of University of California (1976). A young man from India, Prosenjit Poddar, enrolled at the University of California, Berkeley (UC Berkeley) to study naval architecture. In 1968, Poddar met another UC Berkeley student, Tatiana Tarasoff, at a folk dancing class and became smitten. Eventually, Poddar's interest in Tarasoff devolved into an unhealthy obsession and led to stalking. When Poddar told his counselor, a psychologist at UC Berkeley's student health center, about his plans to kill Tarasoff, the psychologist attempted to have Poddar civilly committed. Campus police responded, and Poddar was briefly detained. He was subsequently released after police determined that he was rational and had changed his attitude. Furthermore, the therapist's supervisor reprimanded him for attempting to have Poddar committed and violating his confidentiality and ordered no further action. Tarasoff was thus never alerted to Poddar's threat and was stabbed to death at her parents' home not long afterward.

A lengthy court battle ensued, and the California Supreme Court made two rulings. In 1974, the court ruled that mental health professionals have a duty to warn foreseeable victims, and in 1976, the court ruled that mental health professionals have a duty to protect the foreseeable victim(s) of a dangerous patient. Specifically, the court wrote that

> When a therapist determines, or pursuant to the standards of his profession should determine, that his patient presents a serious danger of violence to another, he incurs an obligation to use reasonable care to protect the intended victim against such danger. The discharge of this duty may require the therapist to take one or more of various steps, depending upon the nature of the case. Thus it may call for him to warn the intended victim or others likely to apprise the victim of the danger, to notify the police, or to take whatever other steps are reasonably necessary under the circumstances. (Tarasoff v. Regents of University of California 1976)

Justice Matthew O. Tobriner notably opined, "The protective privilege ends where the public peril begins." In 1985, California became the first state to enact a statute to codify mental health professionals' *Tarasoff* obligations. Although many states followed in enacting *Tarasoff* statutes, the statutes vary when clarifying this obligation to address potentially dangerous individuals (Kachigian and Felthous 2004). Mental health providers should be familiar with their individual state's *Tarasoff* statute.

At a minimum, the 1976 *Tarasoff* ruling indicated that protective measures include warning the intended victim and possibly informing law enforcement; in some circumstances, mental health professionals are legally obligated to warn the intended victim (Felthous 2006). For example, California Civil Code 43.92 outlines that psychotherapists may be liable "if the patient has communicated to the psychotherapist a serious threat of physical violence against a reasonably identifiable victim or victims" (California Code, Civil Code 2012). The statute states further that the psychotherapist is not liable when he or she "discharges his or her duty to protect by making reasonable efforts to communicate the threat to the victim or victims and to a law enforcement agency" (California Code, Civil Code 2012). State laws regarding therapists' duty to protect have expanded in some jurisdictions during the 40-plus years since the final *Tarasoff* ruling and have extended to broad classes of victims (e.g., coworkers, law enforcement officers, persons of a particular religious or ethnic background) and the public at large as in the cases of Lipari v. Sears, Roebuck and Co. (1980) and Volk v. Demeerleer (2014). In sum, school mental health providers are legally required to break confidentiality when a threat to the safety of other students and, depending on local jurisdiction, the public at large arises.

Developmental Considerations in the Threat Assessment Process

In this subsection, we review approaches to performing threat assessments of students at the elementary, middle, and high school levels (Figure 8–3). It is important to note that a child's developmental level is not always commensurate with his or her age or physical appearance. Thus, evaluators should be prepared to modify their assessments on the basis of the developmental level of evaluees. In general, it is best to begin with open-ended questions when interviewing students making the threats, victims, and witnesses.

Threat Assessment Process Applied to Elementary School Students

Young students may be frightened during an interview with an administrator or other school official. Younger students may also have a difficult time understanding the extent of their actions or precipitating events or may shut down for fear of getting in trouble. Rapport is an important part of any interview, and evaluators should take steps to ensure a student's comfort whenever possible. For instance, acknowledging the understandable fear or apprehension that a student may be experiencing or offering an opportunity to go for a walk or get a drink of water can go a long way in making students feel comfortable.

Elementary school students sometimes struggle to describe complex events, so it may be easier for them to demonstrate what occurred by using small dolls or by drawing pictures. It is also important for evalu-

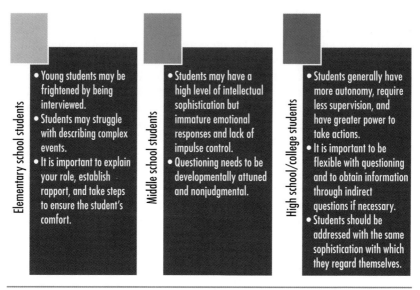

Elementary school students
- Young students may be frightened by being interviewed.
- Students may struggle with describing complex events.
- It is important to explain your role, establish rapport, and take steps to ensure the student's comfort.

Middle school students
- Students may have a high level of intellectual sophistication but immature emotional responses and lack of impulse control.
- Questioning needs to be developmentally attuned and nonjudgmental.

High school/college students
- Students generally have more autonomy, require less supervision, and have greater power to take actions.
- It is important to be flexible with questioning and to obtain information through indirect questions if necessary.
- Students should be addressed with the same sophistication with which they regard themselves.

FIGURE 8–3. Threat assessment considerations in different populations.

ators to be mindful of potentially reexposing students to traumatic events during the interview process, and they should avoid pushing students beyond their limits. If the threats or violent behavior associated with threats are at a level where criminal charges might be filed, evaluators are advised to inform the child's parents and law enforcement in order to represent the best interests of all parties involved rather than attempting to get the story on their own. See Appendix A at the end of the book for suggestions and sample questions that provide a guide for evaluators who wish to obtain information regarding threats from students who are developmentally at the grade school level.

Threat Assessment Process Applied to Middle School Students

Middle school is a challenging time marked by having multiple teachers, increased academic demands, a reshuffling of peer alliances, and puberty. Developmentally, middle school students are trying their hand at separating from parents or caretakers and seeking a place to fit in among peers. Further complicating matters, the very act of seeking help in response to threats during middle school can be tantamount to "snitching" in some situations. For some students, middle school can be a time characterized by loneliness, ostracism or rejection, anxiety, depression, and suicidality. Needless to say, middle school can be overwhelming. From a clinician's standpoint, middle school students can present a particular challenge because they can have a high level of intellectual sophistication coupled with immature emotional responses and lack of impulse control. See Appendix B for suggestions and sample questions that provide a guide for evaluators who wish to obtain information regarding threats from students who are developmentally at the middle school level.

Threat Assessment Process Applied to High School or College Students

High school and college students generally have more autonomy, require less supervision, and have more opportunity to act on threats than do younger students. They are better able to obtain items, from food to guns, and thus have greater power to take actions as they become more independent. See Appendix C for suggestions and sample questions that provide a guide for evaluators who wish to obtain information regarding threats from students who are developmentally at the high school or college level.

Case Vignette *(continued)*

During his evaluation, Justin explains that he has been living with his mother for the past 3 years since the death of his father in a car accident. He adds that at one point his uncle stayed with the family, but his uncle was often physically abusive toward Justin and his mother when he drank alcohol, which occurred frequently. When asked, Justin indicates that child protective services has never been involved with his family. He adds that since his uncle left the home, he has had difficulty sleeping, often waking up with bad dreams of violence. Although he had been previously social with peers at school, Justin began to grow increasingly isolated from former friends and has not remained in contact with any peers since he was removed from his regular high school. Justin describes his mood as "angry, irritated" and states that he does not recall the last time he felt happy. He denies ever thinking about suicide or attempting to harm or kill himself. He reports no alcohol or drug use.

When asked about his daily routine, Justin reports that he is home alone for most of the day while his mother is at work. He states that he spends most of the day on his computer. When asked about what he does on the computer, he says that he watches old footage he found online of past school shooters. He estimates that he spends approximately 3 hours each day watching and rewatching the footage. During other hours of the day, he says, he is researching methods to bomb his school.

Justin's mother states that she is surprised by what Justin has said. She notes that he has never disclosed any violent plans before. She confirms that Justin's uncle was violent with the family when he was around but that he is now living in his own apartment. She describes Justin as more withdrawn and isolated over the past year but says that he does not appear overly sad or depressed. She states that she does not

TABLE 8–5.   **Justin's risk factors and plans for addressing them**

Risk factor	Plan
Imminent danger to others	Refer Justin for psychiatric hospitalization, inform school administration of threats, and contact mother's boyfriend and local law enforcement agency regarding threats (*Tarasoff* duty)
Mental health symptoms	Perform a full psychiatric evaluation to determine a mental health diagnosis and treatment plan (e.g., level of community mental health services needed, psychotropic medication, therapy)
Possible access to weapons	Involve local law enforcement to evaluate Justin's access to firearms and explosive material
Academic decline	Justin's mother should request Individualized Education Program evaluation to determine if Justin is eligible for special education services
Ongoing violence risk	A qualified mental health evaluator could request formal risk assessment using appropriate risk assessment instruments
Child maltreatment	Report alleged physical abuse perpetrated by Justin's uncle to local child welfare agency

have any firearms but that Justin could possibly access firearms from local relatives. She reports that Justin does not receive any special education services, but she has been concerned about his recent poor performance in school. She explains that he has been in therapy over the past few months because of his decline in academics and that he has recently started taking an antidepressant medication.

As a mental health professional, you are concerned that Justin's decline and recent violent ideation are related to a mental health condition such as a trauma-related disorder or depressive disorder. Given his statements, symptoms, and behaviors, he meets criteria for involuntary psychiatric hospitalization as a danger to others due to his mental health. You identify preliminary risk factors and an immediate plan as shown in Table 8–5.

Conclusion

The immediate objective of the threat assessment is to clarify whether the threat is truly meant to harm (physically or emotionally) another person and the likelihood of the alleged perpetrator acting on the threat. Multiple aspects (e.g., motivation, precipitating events, level of planning) should be considered in the assessment. It is generally more concerning when a number of different variables are interconnected and point toward acting on a threat.

If the threat is judged to be transient in nature (not serious, no real harm planned or intended, not feasible), then the threat may be dealt with quickly, and school resumes. If the threat is substantive or if the factors fueling the threat remain active such that the likelihood of subsequent threats or incidents persists, then the next stage, the risk assessment, described in Chapter 9, is appropriate.

Key Points

- *Threats* are specific statements or actions indicating an intent to harm.

- *Risk* is the ongoing ability and capacity of a person to carry out his or her intentions to harm. Violence risk refers to factors that make a person more or less likely to engage in violent behavior.

- A comprehensive school team composed of administrators, teachers, mental health clinicians, and law enforcement is critical in responding to serious threats.

- In most jurisdictions across the United States, mental health providers are either required or permitted to break confidentiality in order to warn or protect third parties from violent patients.

- According to the Safe School Initiative, most incidents of targeted school violence are planned with others having advanced knowledge of the attacker's intentions and behaving in ways that draw concern from others.

Clinical Pearls

Findings from the Safe School Initiative included that most studied incidents of targeted violence were planned, that other people had advance knowledge of the attacker's ideas or plans, and that most of the attackers were behaving in ways that caused prior concern from others.

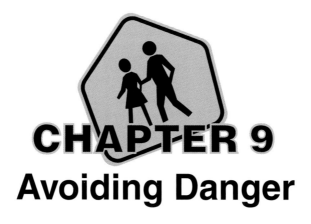

CHAPTER 9
Avoiding Danger

The Principles of Violence Risk Assessment

Anne B. McBride, M.D.

Arany Uthayakumar, B.A.

Michael B. Kelly, M.D.

A ship in harbor is safe, but that is not what ships are built for.

John Augustus Shedd

Case Vignette

Rene is a 15-year-old girl with a reported history of gang affiliation. She has no juvenile justice record or known history of violence. Rene was attacked outside her school by three young women who do not attend the school. The school security officer who broke up the altercation stated that Rene's three assailants threatened to "come back for [her]." Rene responded to the attackers by telling them that she will "find you and stab all of you, you'll see!" Rene was provided medical attention then met with school staff and law enforcement. Despite the threats directed at her attackers, Rene says that she does not know her attackers and that she has no idea why she was targeted.

In this chapter, we focus on the nuts and bolts of conducting a violence risk assessment. We review the principles involved in violence risk assessment in youth and the use of standardized instruments developed to evaluate for youth violence risk. We then provide an overview of conducting the evaluation as well as the specific features of the violence risk assessment.

Overview of Violence Risk Assessment in Youth

In general, mental health professionals are not particularly accurate at predicting violence. Although most studies "suggest that mental health professionals have at least a moderate ability to predict violence and that their predictions are significantly more accurate than chance" (Borum 1996, p. 946), mental health professionals are still prone to making incorrect predictions, most commonly making false positives errors (Otto 1992). Given these limitations, assessing an individual's *risk* of future violence is much more meaningful. The purpose of a violence risk assessment is to identify risk and protective factors that raise or lower the youth's risk of future violence so that a targeted plan can be created to mitigate that risk of future violence.

Risk factors are typically thought of as being either static or dynamic. *Static* risk factors are those that are not subject to intervention and tend to be historical, such as an individual's past violent behaviors, history of maltreatment, or early exposure to domestic violence. Although these risk factors should be considered in formulating an individual's overall risk of future violence, they may be less informative when developing a risk response plan. *Dynamic* factors are those that are modifiable, such as substance use, symptoms of mental illness, and access to weapons. These are the types of factors that are most useful to identify and incorporate into a plan to lower the risk of violence by addressing factors that can be changed.

A unique aspect of violence risk assessment in youth is its dynamism. That is, youth tend to be quite different at age 8 years compared with age 15 years compared with age 25 years. Youth is a time of significant fluidity and development that makes addressing dynamic risk factors supremely important. Additionally, optimizing protective factors can substantially impact a youth's development and reduce future violence risk. An adequate risk assessment should include the risk and protective factors present or notably absent and a specific plan to address each factor moving forward.

Broadly, there are three major approaches to violence risk assessment. *Clinical judgment*, or an unstructured and purely clinical approach to assessing dangerousness, involves one side of the spectrum of risk assessment. Mental health professionals use this approach frequently such as in emergency or other clinical settings where acute safety risk is determined. Early studies of the accuracy of using clinical judgment alone to predict dangerousness were discouraging. However, more recent studies suggest that clinicians can distinguish violent individuals from nonviolent individuals with a "modest, better-than-chance level of accuracy" (Mossman 1994, p. 790).

Actuarial assessments are the other extreme on the spectrum of violence risk assessment and involve formulas used to predict concrete risk of future violence based on a set of risk factors known to be associated with recidivism. This involves compiling data that yield a value for future risk where, in general, there is a linear relationship between the numerical score and final risk estimate. Literature has suggested that statistical formulas generally perform as well as or better than clinical judgments (Borum et al. 2006). However, actuarial assessments are generally based on static factors and therefore are not as helpful when attempting to modify risks for individuals.

The third type of violence risk assessment is known as *structured professional judgment*. Tools for this assessment type involve structured guides that specifically identify known risk factors from the literature and guide the evaluator to systematically review checklists of these factors, determining each factor's presence or absence and relevance in order to formulate a thorough risk assessment and final judgment. This review does not yield final numerical scores and is meant instead to assist in the development of a thoughtful and empirically based formulation of an individual's overall risk for future violence. Importantly, these instruments can provide context for an individual's risk level by allowing the evaluator to explore the etiology leading to violent or threatening behaviors. Moreover, given that the ultimate goal of a risk assessment should be to *prevent* rather than predict future violence, structured professional judgment instruments assist the evaluator in identifying dynamic and modifiable risk factors as well as present and absent protective factors. These factors then can be highlighted to generate highly specific management and intervention plans aimed at reducing the individual's future risk of violence. These tools can also be used over time to measure changes in level of risk as dynamic factors are subsequently modified.

Some risk assessment instruments that have been developed for youth are based on the risk-need-responsivity (RNR) model proposed by Andrews and colleagues as core principles to inform effective programming in a criminal or juvenile justice program (Andrews et al. 1990). In this model, the *risk* principle focuses on *who* should be treated, emphasizing that studies indicate that intensive services should be directed at the higher-risk offenders and minimized with low-risk offenders, where resources would be wasted. Additionally, lower-risk individuals may actually be at increased risk to reoffend when exposed to higher-risk individuals. The *need* principle addresses *what* should be treated and can be implemented by using formal risk assessment tools to identify needs such as criminogenic dynamic risk factors (factors leading to criminal behavior) for treatment purposes. The *responsivity* principle includes providing treatment using a style and mode that are individualized and responsive to the offender's learning style and ability (Andrews and Bonta 2010).

Juvenile Violence Risk Assessment Instruments

The use of structured risk assessments such as actuarial measures or structured professional judgment tools has been shown to lead to more accurate risk assessments when compared with using unstructured clinical judgment alone (Ægisdóttir et al. 2006). Although multiple assessment instruments are available for youth violence, the three tools that have acquired the most substantial empirical support are the Structured Assessment of Violence Risk in Youth (SAVRY), the Youth Level of Service/Case Management Inventory 2.0 (YLS/CMI 2.0), and the Hare Psychopathy Checklist: Youth Version (PCL:YV). A meta-analysis involving 8,746 youth looking at the predictive accuracy of these three instruments showed that they performed equally well (Olver et al. 2009). All three assessment tools were significantly correlated with the prediction of general, nonviolent, and violent recidivism.

Of note, formal violence risk assessment instruments are intended to evaluate general violence risk rather than targeted violence in which a youth poses a threat to a specific person or entity (e.g., school). For example, a youth may not have many risk factors for general violence that would be identified on formal risk assessment but still may pose a high risk to the intended target. Therefore, these tools are best used as an adjunct to the overall risk assessment. They are especially helpful for identifying treatable or modifiable risk factors when developing a safety plan and should not be used as the only component of a violence risk evaluation.

Structured Assessment of Violence Risk in Youth

The SAVRY is a guide for violence risk assessment in youth between ages 12 and 18 years based on the structured professional judgment model that systematically reviews risk factors with known associations to violent offending on the basis of existing scientific and professional literature. The tool can be used with either male or female youth and can be cautiously used in youth who fall slightly outside the targeted age window. The authors' goal in developing the SAVRY was to develop an instrument that is systematic, empirically grounded, developmentally informed, treatment oriented, flexible, and practical. The SAVRY guides the evaluator through 24 risk items (historical, social/contextual, and individual/clinical) and 6 protective factors based on empirical research concerning adolescent development and violence in youth. The evaluator rates each risk item as low, moderate, or high and each protective factor as present or absent. The SAVRY does not result in a final numerical score but rather identifies relevant factors to consider when formulating an individual's overall risk for future violence. The SAVRY has demonstrated a moderate to strong relationship with general and violent recidivism (Catchpole and Gretton 2003; Meyers and Schmidt 2008), and research has supported the validity of the SAVRY when used in a juvenile justice context (Lawing et al. 2017) and to predict probation outcomes (Childs et al. 2013).

Youth Level of Service/Case Management Inventory 2.0

The YLS/CMI 2.0 is a standardized actuarial instrument based on the RNR model used to assess risk, need, and responsivity factors in male and female juvenile offenders, as well as to formulate a case plan. The YLS/CMI 2.0 was normed for juvenile offenders ages 12–18 years in both custodial and community settings. Therefore, it would be appropriate to use with youth who have become involved with the juvenile justice system either historically or with their current behavior. The authors of the YLS/CMI 2.0 indicate that individuals using this instrument may include probation officers, youth workers, psychologists, and social workers.

The YLS/CMI 2.0 includes rating 42 risk items that have been identified as the most predictive of juvenile criminal behavior across 8 categories: prior and current offenses or dispositions, family circumstances and parenting, education and employment, peer relations, substance abuse, leisure and recreation, personality and behavior, and attitudes and orientation. Total risk/need scores are calculated numerically in all broad categories as well as overall, yielding ratings of low, moderate, high, or very high. The tool provides for the assessment of other needs and special considerations before a determination of final risk/need. The YLS/CMI 2.0 also includes a professional override when considering all factors relevant to an individual case.

This instrument can aid the evaluator in making program or placement decisions regarding supervision level needed and provides guidance in forming a case management plan and review (Hoge and Andrews 2011). Bechtel et al. (2007) studied 4,482 juvenile offenders in both custodial and community settings and found that the YLS/CMI 2.0 predicted recidivism (receiving any type of conviction or commitment) in both settings. A recent report for the juvenile probation system in the state of Nebraska involving 6,158 juvenile probationers, just over a third of whom were female, found "strong evidence for the validity" of the YLS/CMI 2.0, with "no evidence for disparate impact in predicting outcomes due to either sex of the youth or race/ethnicity of the youth" (Wiener et al. 2017, p. 64). Data regarding the apparent lack of racial bias inherent in the YLS/CMI 2.0 are supported by a recent field study involving both the YLS/CMI 2.0 and SAVRY in which neither "differentially predict[ed] reoffending as a function of race" (Perrault et al. 2017, p. 664).

Hare Psychopathy Checklist: Youth Version

In 1941, Hervey Cleckley published work describing traits of a psychopath such as superficial charm, untruthfulness, and lack of remorse. In 1980, Robert Hare operationalized the concept of the psychopath and created the Hare Psychopathy Checklist (PCL), which was an instrument designed to quantify the construct of psychopathy (Hare 1980). Hare outlined the characteristics described by Cleckley such as callousness, remorselessness, and egocentricity and combined these traits with behavioral problems stemming from such deficits, such as chronic instability, antisocial behaviors, and the maintenance of a socially deviant lifestyle. The PCL-Revised (PCL-R) is not the only instrument designed to quantify psychopathy but is the one most often used for this construct. Although this instrument is not a risk assessment, substantial research has supported that the PCL-R is strongly related to future violence and violent offending, which is why it is included in most risk assessments.

The construct of juvenile psychopathy, which describes a similar characterological disorder consisting of such traits as glibness, charm, lack of empathy, lack of emotion, impulsiveness, and irresponsibility, is more controversial. Some researchers maintain that labeling a youth as having psychopathic traits is stigmatizing and misleading, given that youth are still developing their identities throughout adolescence. Additionally, juvenile psychopathy instruments have not been shown to reliably predict recidivism in adolescent females and ethnic minorities (Edens et al. 2007). However, increasing evidence supports that juvenile psychopathy is predictive of general and violent recidivism. Therefore, measuring psychopathy in youth can be a useful component in a broader violence risk assessment.

The PCL: Youth Version (PCL:YV) was adapted from the PCL-R to measure psychopathic traits in youth ages 12–18 years. The PCL:YV was not developed to be used as a violence risk instrument but rather was developed so that researchers could learn about adolescent psychopathy, improve understanding in factors related to the development of psychopathy, and evaluate the predictive validity of psychopathic features in juvenile offenders (Forth et al. 2003). The PCL:YV manual specifies that "The PCL:YV should not be the sole criterion used to make decisions about a youth or for dispositions within the mental health and criminal justice system" (Forth et al. 2003, p. 4). The PCL:YV consists of 20 items used to measure the interpersonal, affective, antisocial, and behavioral features of psychopathy using multidomain and multisource information. Although a total score is calculated, cut scores for clinical diagnoses of psychopathy are not provided. Evaluators administering the PCL:YV should possess specific professional requirements, including adequate training and experience in the use of the PCL:YV (Forth et al. 2003).

Asscher et al. (2011) performed a meta-analysis of 53 studies involving the PCL:YV that included 10,073 juvenile participants and found a moderate association between psychopathy and delinquency, general recidivism, and violent recidivism. Specifically, callous-unemotional traits and impulsiveness were both strongly associated with delinquency, and impulsivity was somewhat more strongly associated with recidivism (Asscher et al. 2011). The PCL:YV requires specific training and takes considerable time to complete because it involves an extensive interview and expansive record review. Therefore, researchers have also examined the role of shorter screens in measuring psychopathy. For example, recent research has indicated the validity of the abbreviated 18-item version of the self-report Youth Psychopathic Traits Inventory–Short version (Gillen et al. 2017; Vahl et al. 2014).

Conducting a Developmentally Attuned Risk Assessment

The risk assessment can be integrated into a more familiar mental health evaluation, particularly if done by the school's mental health clinician or by an outside mental health provider. An outline for the mental health evaluation, with additions for evaluating the threat(s) and persisting risks, is as follows:

1. Identifying information (e.g., age, gender identification, living situation, grade level)
2. History of current illness (e.g., current symptoms, impacts on functioning with peers and family and at school)
   a. Prominent (most impairing) symptoms
   b. Substance use and exposure
   c. Trauma exposures

3. Past mental health history (e.g., previous treaters and treatments, treatment adherence, hospitalizations, suicidal thinking and behavior)
   a. Medications
   b. Psychological and neuropsychological testing
4. Past medical history (e.g., significant illnesses, hospitalizations, surgeries, medications for non–mental health conditions, allergies)
5. Developmental and social history (e.g., attainment of speech, motor, and social milestones; transitions to school; separations from caregivers; living environment; neighborhood; educational history; peer relationships; parental/caregiver support)
6. Family history (e.g., maternal, paternal, siblings with mental health conditions, substance use, criminal behaviors)
7. Mental status examination (e.g., appearance, speech, mood and affect, sensorium, thought process and content)
8. Risk assessment (integrating threat assessment with the mental health evaluation and a focus on risk and protective factors and addressing those factors later in the treatment recommendations)
9. Formulation
10. Treatment recommendations

In addition to a standard mental health evaluation, violence risk assessments include focused attention on and exploration of specific topics, including the current threat or violent event warranting the assessment, the individual's history of previous violent behavior, weapons history, exposure to violence and trauma, conduct problems, substance use, psychiatric history, and other risk factors associated with future violence (Figure 9–1).

Current Threat or Violent Event

The mental health evaluation should include a thorough exploration of the precipitating event leading to the assessment. This includes questions about intent and motivation to engage in violence, planning that has occurred, steps that have been taken toward committing the violent act, and intended targets of violence, including individuals or entities. The evaluator should obtain information about when plans were formulated and when the individual took further steps, if indicated. The evaluator should also explore the individual's perceived goals and ideas about the outcome and consequences if the act is carried out.

Past History of Violent Behaviors

An individual's past behaviors are often the best predictor of future behavior. Therefore, in a risk assessment it is essential to gather informa-

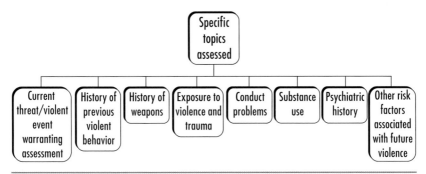

FIGURE 9–1. **Topics explored in violence risk assessments.**

tion about the student's history of violent behavior. Often, this will require obtaining collateral information (e.g., family, victim, professionals, documentation). An evaluation of the student may include questions about anger management; onset of violent behavior; frequency of violence; magnitude of violence; and the individual's thoughts and feelings prior to, at the time of, and following the violent act.

Weapons History

Most murders committed by juveniles involve the use of firearms (Office of Juvenile Justice and Delinquency Prevention 2016). Evaluating for access to weapons and past use of weapons is an especially important component in the risk assessment. This includes questions regarding past exposure to weapons (e.g., firearms, knives, explosives), past use of weapons, attitudes toward firearms and other weapons, carrying of weapons, and current access to weapons (at home or accessible by other means).

Exposure to Violence and Trauma

Exposure to violence and maltreatment or trauma are significant risk factors associated with violence in general (Borum et al. 2006). A risk assessment should include questions regarding the individual's exposure to both current and past violence at home, in the community, and within his or her peer group. Exploring the individual's own history of sustained trauma or maltreatment is also important. In some cases, maltreatment by caretakers (physical abuse, sexual abuse, emotional abuse, or neglect) may be ongoing or may have not been previously reported to child protective services. In such cases, immediate referral to child welfare agencies is necessary.

Conduct Problems

Delinquent behaviors, both violent and nonviolent, are associated with risk of future violence (Borum et al. 2006). A review of behaviors that violate the rights of others or other age-appropriate social norms is necessary. DSM-5 (American Psychiatric Association 2013) lists 15 behaviors associated with conduct disorder. See Table 9–1 for a list of possible conduct problems that should be explored. Additional traits to explore include indicators of lack of remorse or guilt, callousness or lack of empathy, lack of concern about performance, and shallow or deficient affect. The DSM-5 conduct disorder diagnosis includes a *with limited prosocial emotions* specifier requiring that a youth display at least two of the following characteristics over at least a year in multiple relationships and settings: lack of remorse or guilt, callouness or lack of empathy, lack of concern about performance, and shallow or deficient affect. These characteristics are often referred to as "callous-unemotional traits" in youth violence literature. Youth with callous-unemotional traits often have more severe conduct problems and violence that can become resistant to intervention as the youth ages (for a relevant review of early identification and treatment of antisocial behavior, see Frick 2016). Additional areas of focus in a youth with possible conduct problems include his or her attitudes toward criminal behavior, typical responses to conflict, and peer relationships (e.g., associating with negative, delinquent peers versus positive, prosocial peers).

Substance Use

Use of substances, particularly if currently being misused, is often associated with violence (Steadman et al. 1998; Swanson et al. 1990). The evaluator should obtain a thorough substance use history that includes past and current use of alcohol or illicit substances such as cannabis, stimulants, opioids, and hallucinogens and misuse of prescription pills. Questions should cover longevity of use, frequency of use, indicators of problematic or compulsive use, and access to substances. Inquiring about the relationship between substance use and past violence or aggression may also be informative.

Psychiatric History

In addition to standard questions about an individual's psychiatric history as reviewed in the section "Conducting a Developmentally Attuned Risk Assessment," other specific foci can be queries about current or active psychiatric symptoms (e.g., depression, mania, anxiety, psychosis, trauma-related symptoms), current treatment, and past relation-

TABLE 9–1. Behaviors associated with conduct disorder

According to DSM-5 diagnostic criteria, behaviors associated with conduct disorder include the following:

Aggression to people and animals

1. Often bullies, threatens, or intimidates others.

2. Often initiates physical fights.

3. Has used a weapon that can cause serious physical harm to others (e.g., a bat, brick, broken bottle, knife, gun).

4. Has been physically cruel to people.

5. Has been physically cruel to animals.

6. Has stolen while confronting a victim (e.g., mugging, purse snatching, extortion, armed robbery).

7. Has forced someone into sexual activity.

Destruction of property

8. Has deliberately engaged in fire setting with the intention of causing serious damage.

9. Has deliberately destroyed others' property (other than by fire setting).

Deceitfulness or theft

10. Has broken into someone else's house, building, or car.

11. Often lies to obtain goods or favors or to avoid obligations (i.e., "cons" others).

12. Has stolen items of nontrivial value without confronting a victim (e.g., shoplifting, but without breaking and entering; forgery).

Serious violations of rules

13. Often stays out at night despite parental prohibitions, beginning before age 13 years.

14. Has run away from home overnight at least twice while living in the parental or parental surrogate home, or once without returning for a lengthy period.

15. Is often truant from school, beginning before age 13 years.

ships between psychiatric symptoms and violent behaviors or ideation. Additionally, given that impulsivity and history of attention-deficit/ hyperactivity disorder are associated with youth violence specifically (Borum et al. 2006), the evaluator should inquire about these symptoms, diagnoses, and past and current treatment.

Other Risk Factors Associated With Future Violence

As discussed here and in Chapter, 8, "Hostile Intent," there are multiple risk factors associated with future violence or targeted violence for specific individuals. The evaluator should be aware of risk factors that may be unique to the individual and explore these factors accordingly.

Collateral Interviews and Other Sources of Information

In addition to interviewing the individual student, obtaining collateral sources of information is typically necessary when conducting a risk assessment. This may include collateral interviews with parents or caregivers, teachers, school officials, mental health providers, and others. A review of records may also be illuminating and may provide corroborating or refuting data. Records may include police reports, mental health records, educational records, disciplinary records, and child protective service records.

Risk Formulation

Use of the risk assessment instruments occurs following an interview with the youth and a review of collateral interviews and other sources of information. Evaluators should be familiar with the specific instrument they might use prior to conducting an evaluation to help structure the type of information applicable in a violence risk assessment. In general, a comprehensive psychiatric or psychological evaluation should overlap with information important to review in a risk assessment. When all the available information is gathered, the evaluator then reviews the specific risk assessment. For example, when the SAVRY is applied, the evaluator will then review each of the 24 risk factors and 6 protective factors identified in the SAVRY in a systematic manner to help structure the risk formulation.

In the risk formulation, the evaluator summarizes the individual's risk and protective factors in a concise manner, describing the etiology leading to the current level of risk of future violence. In this section of the evaluation, the evaluator provides a statement to indicate whether the individual's risk of future violence is low, moderate, or high, along with an explanation for how the evaluator arrived at this conclusion. This is also an opportunity to summarize protective factors or risk factors that are notably absent; these may be strengths used to lower the youth's risk for future violence.

Treatment Plan

The main goal of a violence risk assessment should be to formulate a risk management or treatment plan once the level of risk is identified. The treatment plan in a risk assessment involves identifying the dynamic risk factors present for the individual that contribute to his or her risk of violence. It also provides a specific plan for intervention to modify these risk factors in order to ultimately lower the risk of future violence. For example, a plan may include statements such as the following:

1. Active psychotic symptoms—refer for immediate mental health treatment through emergency psychiatric services for treatment and management of symptoms
2. Cannabis use—provide linkage to substance abuse treatment program
3. Access to firearms in home—work with local law enforcement to confiscate or secure weaponry

Case Vignette *(continued)*

School officials call Rene's parents, who advise her to be forthcoming with school officials and law enforcement. Rene says that the young women who assaulted her are affiliated with a local street gang, adding that one of the young women is now dating her ex-boyfriend. Rene says that she knows all three of her assailants, that they are known to use drugs, and that two of them have been arrested previously for assault. Rene's parents insist that their daughter divulge the names of her attackers, and she eventually complies. School officials and law enforcement conclude that the threat to Rene is serious and credible. Police are dispatched to the residences of her attackers, and all three are taken into custody.

Rene's parents get their daughter to divulge that she has a knife at home that she keeps for protection, which is handed over to police. Despite Rene's lack of criminal history, school officials and law enforcement agree that steps must be taken to reduce the likelihood of Rene being the victim or perpetrator of targeted violence. Rene is referred for a psychological evaluation. She is also referred to a local gang rescue program that includes counselors who are themselves former gang members.

Rene's psychological evaluation reveals that she was sexually assaulted by an adult male neighbor when she was 8 years old and that the perpetrator is currently serving time in state prison. Rene is ultimately diagnosed with generalized anxiety disorder, a cannabis use disorder of moderate severity, and oppositional defiant disorder of moderate severity. It is also determined that Rene has met full criteria for posttraumatic stress disorder (PTSD) in the past and continues to experience some PTSD symptoms. Rene is referred for trauma-focused cognitive-behavioral therapy and substance use counseling with regular urine toxicology screening. Rene's parents are referred to a parenting coach who will help them create, maintain, and enforce a home behavior plan. Rene is also encouraged to join her school's cross-country team and begins attending practice regularly.

Conclusion

In summary, a violence risk assessment is typically conducted by a mental health professional who has experience working with youth and youth violence. The assessment includes a standard mental health evaluation with specific areas explored in as much detail as is relevant to the risk of violence that is being assessed. Standardized instruments that assess specifically for youth violence risk yield more accurate assessments than do other instruments. The assessment should include a summary formulation and detailed plan for intervention targeting modifiable or dynamic risk factors.

Key Points

- Violence risk assessment identifies risk and protective factors so that a targeted plan can be created to mitigate future violence risk.

- Static, or historical, risk factors cannot be modified by intervention; they include an individual's history of past violence or early experiences with maltreatment.

- Dynamic factors can be modified; examples of dynamic factors include symptoms of mental illness, access to weapons, and substance abuse.

- Structured professional judgment uses a confluence of clinical expertise and structured, research-driven guides to develop thoughtful and empirical evaluations of future violence risk.

- Actuarial approaches use static (historical) risk factors to generate a score indicating the likelihood of future violence.

Clinical Pearls

Collateral sources of information (e.g., caretakers, family members) are important when determining a youth's access to weapons.

Substance use magnifies violence risk.

References

Ægisdóttir S, White MJ, Spengler PM, et al: The meta-analysis of clinical judgment project: fifty-six years of accumulated research on clinical versus statistical prediction. Counseling Psychologist 34(3):341–382, 2006

American Psychiatric Association: Diagnostic and Statistical Manual of Mental Disorders, 5th Edition. Arlington, VA, American Psychiatric Association, 2013

Andrews DA, Bonta J: Rehabilitating criminal justice policy and practice. Psychol Public Policy Law 16(1):39–55, 2010

Andrews DA, Bonta J, Hoge RD: Classification for effective rehabilitation: rediscovering psychology. Crim Justice Behav 17(1):19–52, 1990

Asscher JJ, van Vugt ES, Stams GJ, et al: The relationship between juvenile psychopathic traits, delinquency and (violent) recidivism: a meta-analysis. J Child Psychol Psychiatry 52(11):1134–1143, 2011 21599664

Bechtel K, Lowenkamp CT, Latessa E: Assessing the risk of re-offending for juvenile offenders using the Youth Level of Service/Case Management Inventory. J Offender Rehabil 45(3–4):85–108, 2007

Borum R: Improving the clinical practice of violence risk assessment: technology, guidelines, and training. Am Psychol 51(9):945–956, 1996 8819363

Borum R, Bartel P, Forth A: Structured Assessment of Violence Risk in Youth Professional Manual. Lutz, FL, Psychological Assessment Resources, 2006

Catchpole REH, Gretton HM: The predictive validity of risk assessment with violent young offenders: a 1-year examination of criminal outcome. Crim Justice Behav 30(6):688–708, 2003

Childs KK, Ryals J Jr, Frick PJ, et al: Examining the validity of the Structured Assessment of Violence Risk In Youth (SAVRY) for predicting probation outcomes among adjudicated juvenile offenders. Behav Sci Law 31(2):256–270, 2013 23606362

Edens JF, Campbell JS, Weir JM: Youth psychopathy and criminal recidivism: a meta-analysis of the psychopathy checklist measures. Law Hum Behav 31(1):53–75, 2007 17019617

Forth AE, Kossen DS, Hare RD: Hare Psychopathy Checklist: Youth Version Technical Manual. North Tonawanda, NY, Multi-Health Systems, 2003

Frick PJ: Early identification and treatment of antisocial behavior. Pedatr Clin North Am 63(5):861–871, 2016 27565364

Gillen CT, MacDougall EA, Forth AE, et al: Validity of the youth psychopathic traits inventory–short version in justice-involved and at-risk adolescents. Assessment 2017 28397535 Epub ahead of print

Hare RD: A research scale for the assessment of psychopathy in criminal populations. Pers Individ Dif 1(2):111–119, 1980

Hoge RD, Andrews DA: Youth Level of Service/Case Management Inventory 2.0 User's Manual. North Tonawanda, NY, Multi-Health Systems, 2011

Lawing K, Childs KK, Frick PJ, et al: Use of structured professional judgment by probation officers to assess risk for recidivism in adolescent offenders. Psychol Assess 29(6):652–663, 2017 28594209

Meyers JR, Schmidt F: Predictive validity of the structured assessment for violence risk in youth (SAVRY) with juvenile offenders. Crim Justice Behav 35(3):344–355, 2008

Mossman D: Assessing predictions of violence: being accurate about accuracy. J Consult Clin Psychol 62(4):783–792, 1994 7962882

Office of Juvenile Justice and Delinquency Prevention: OJJDP Statistical Briefing Book. Washington, DC, Office of Juvenile Justice and Delinquency Prevention, 2016. Available at: www.ojjdp.gov/ojstatbb/offenders/qa03103.asp?qaDate=2016. Accessed March 30, 2019.

Otto R: The prediction of dangerous behavior: a review and analysis of "second generation" research. Forensic Reports 5:103–133, 1992

Olver ME, Stockdale KC, Warmth S: Risk assessment with young offenders: a meta-analysis of three assessment instruments. Crim Justice Behav 36(4):329–353, 2009

Perrault RT, Vincent GM, Guy LS: Are risk assessments racially biased? Field study of the SAVRY and YLS/CMI in probation. Psychol Assess 29(6):664–678, 2017 28594210

Steadman HJ, Mulvey EP, Monahan J, et al: Violence by people discharged from acute psychiatric inpatient facilities and by others in the same neighborhoods. Arch Gen Psychiatry 55:393–401, 1998 9596041

Swanson JW, Holzer CE 3rd, Ganju VK, et al: Violence and psychiatric disorders in the community: evidence from the Epidemiologic Catchment Area surveys. Hosp Community Psychiatry 41(7):761–770, 1990 2142118

Vahl P, Colins OF, Lodewijks HPB, et al: Psychopathic-like traits in detained adolescents: clinical usefulness of self-report. Eur Child Adolesc Psychiatry 23(8):691–699, 2014 24327266

Wiener RL, Jimenez AC, Petty JT, et al: Predictive Validity of the YLS/CMI as Administered in Nebraska Probation. Lincoln, NE, University of Nebraska Law Psychology Program, 2017

PART III
Interventions

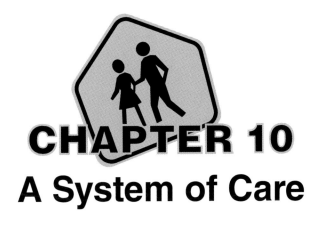

CHAPTER 10
A System of Care

Addressing Aggression and Violence in Schools

Michael B. Kelly, M.D.

Anne B. McBride, M.D.

Ana DiRago, Ph.D.

Arany Uthayakumar, B.A.

The greatness of a community is most accurately measured by the compassionate actions of its members.

Coretta Scott King

Case Vignette

Lorraine is a 17-year-old high school senior who was referred for evaluation after she wrote a short story for English class about a girl who walked into the teacher's lounge and opened fire with a rifle, killing several of her current teachers, who are identified by name in the story. When Lorraine's teacher and other school staff asked her about the story, she maintained eye contact but did not speak.

Lorraine is referred initially to the school counselor. A school administrator shares with the counselor that Lorraine attended a gifted program in middle school and was an A student her freshman and sophomore years. Over the past year and a half, her grades have declined. She was sent to detention a couple of times for drawing in class despite her teachers asking her to put the drawings aside. Lorraine used to have a group of friends but now is a "loner" who has become increasingly withdrawn. Moreover, she dropped out of her debate team junior year and left the National Honor Society because of declining academic performance.

Lorraine's English teacher describes her as a good writer; however, her stories have become "bizarre" and somewhat difficult to follow. The teacher shared that some students have begun to make fun of Lorraine because it appears that she has not been washing her hair and she always wears the same shirt.

The interventions summarized in this chapter focus on the prevention of violence and treatment of individuals at risk for engaging in violent behavior. Preventative interventions can be classified as primary, secondary, or tertiary in nature (Figure 10–1). Primary violence prevention programs aim to reduce the likelihood of violence at the population or school-wide level. Primary prevention programs do not target a particular high-risk group. Secondary prevention programs, on the other hand, are designed for persons who are at an elevated risk for committing acts of violence. An example of secondary prevention is treating underlying depression and attention-deficit/hyperactivity disorder (ADHD) in a student who has made threats of violence. Tertiary prevention is meant to mitigate violence risk in persons with prior histories of violence. Treatment programs designed for juvenile sex offenders exemplify tertiary prevention.

Treatment refers to interventions designed to prevent future violence or treat underlying psychopathology, if present, that is contributing to violent behaviors. Although most violent behavior is not due to a mental illness, as discussed in greater detail in Chapter 7, "Growing Up in Fear," mental health conditions can contribute to violence risk. Moreover, aggression can be a basic part of human life, even healthy in some contexts. Therefore, we do not think of violence as something that can be "cured." Information on the programs described in this chapter and other programs can be found at www.blueprintsprograms.com.

School Services

School counselors often are important members of the treatment team for at-risk youth. They can provide onsite school counseling services and also refer youth for more urgent evaluation if they pose an imminent safety risk to themselves or others.

If there is any indication that a youth may have symptoms (e.g., learning difficulties, emotional problems) that impair his or her ability to benefit from educational services, the youth should be evaluated for special education services. This would occur under the Individuals

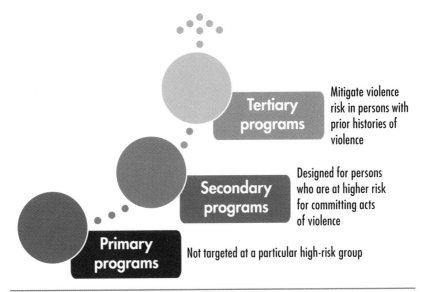

FIGURE 10-1. **Progression of interventions.**

with Disabilities Education Act (IDEA) through an Individualized Education Program (IEP) evaluation. The purpose of the IDEA is "to ensure that all children with disabilities have available to them a free appropriate public education that emphasizes special education and related services designed to meet their unique needs and prepare them for further education, employment and independent living" as well as to ensure that these rights are protected, to assist agencies in the provision of such education, and to assess and ensure effectiveness of the education efforts (Individuals with Disabilities Education Act 2004). If youth have a qualifying disability under IDEA, then they may require special education and additional services through an IEP so that they can appropriately access and benefit from their educational services. Related services for "providing appropriate special education and related services, and aids and supports in the regular classroom, to such children, whenever appropriate" as included under the IDEA are listed in Table 10-1.

Students with disabilities who do not qualify for special education services through an IEP may still qualify for accommodations through Section 504 of the Rehabilitation Act of 1973 (2002). Whereas IDEA is education legislation and the main vehicle for obtaining special education services, Section 504 and Title II of the Americans with Disabilities Act of 1990 (2008) are civil rights statutes that protect individuals with disabilities and apply to all federally funded schools and agencies as well as state and local government services, prohibiting discrimination

TABLE 10–1. Types of related services that may be used in an Individualized Education Program

Transportation

Speech-language pathology and audiology services

Interpreting services

Psychological services

Physical and occupational therapy

Therapeutic recreation

Social work services

School nurse services

Rehabilitation counseling

Orientation and mobility services

Medical services (for evaluation purposes only; not for diagnostic purposes)

on the basis of disability in these settings. Essentially, Section 504 serves to ensure that students with disabilities have the same access to educational services, programs, and activities as their nondisabled peers. Section 504, unlike IDEA, does not allot funding for services. However, Section 504 can be used in practice to obtain reasonable school or classroom accommodations that would prevent discrimination within the school setting. For example, a student with ADHD and poor frustration tolerance may benefit from accommodations that allow him or her to take a 15-minute break from the classroom when upset to "cool off" before returning to the classroom.

In cases where the youth at risk for violence already has an IEP or 504 plan in place, a new event (such as making threats in the school setting) may prompt a reevaluation of special education services or accommodations to consider if the IEP or 504 plan needs to be adjusted or supplemented with additional services. Sometimes the student may benefit from transferring to a different educational setting. In the most extreme cases, this may include a residential setting.

When a student with an IEP behaves in such a way at school that warrants disciplinary action, the student may be suspended without triggering an IEP meeting but with limits of no more than 10 consecutive school days per year. In cases that involve weapons or drugs, the student may have his or her placement changed to an alternative education setting for up to 45 days. In some instances in which behavior warrants disciplinary action that includes more than 10 days of removal or a change in placement, the school will conduct a manifestation determination to determine whether the behavior was a manifestation of the child's disability. If the behavior was not a manifestation of the child's disability, the child can be disciplined as usual. If the behavior was a manifestation of the child's disability, the IEP team must look at the current placement and consider if it is still appropriate in light of the behavior. A behavioral assessment and intervention plan may be indicated. If a child with an IEP is expelled, the school district is required to provide free appropriate public education in another setting. If the child needs residential placement because of behaviors that are a manifestation of his or her disability, the cost is the school district's responsibility. Students are sometimes placed in juvenile detention facilities or jails because of incidents that may or may not be related to on-campus behavior problems. Detained children continue to maintain their IEPs.

Community Services

Mental Health

Many youth require additional services offered through the community, such as in areas of mental health care. Mental health treatment can be provided through private funding (e.g., private insurance, self-pay) or through community-based, county, or state programs and agencies, funded through public sources. In cases involving psychiatric emergencies, in which mental health symptoms are linked to dangerousness (toward others or self), the youth should be evaluated in an emergency setting (e.g., psychiatric crisis center, emergency department) for possible psychiatric hospitalization. Once psychiatric symptoms are stabilized, some youth may benefit from step-down psychiatric services such as partial hospitalization or intensive outpatient programs, where they do not reside in an acute locked psychiatric facility but still benefit from intensive day program services. Ultimately, the youth will be transitioned to outpatient mental health services. This may involve a wide array of service providers, depending on the level of intensity needed. Typically, at a minimum, the youth will have a therapist and, when psychotropic medications are indicated, a child and adolescent psychiatrist on his or her team. Outpatient services may be administered at a mental health clinic, at the school, or at the child's residence.

Substance Use

Substance abuse treatment is also typically accessed adjunctively through the community. If use of illicit substances is suspected, the youth's physician may conduct screening to determine if referral for substance use treatment is indicated. Youth may also directly contact an addiction specialist (e.g., through sources generated through the American Society of Addiction Medicine and the American Academy of Child and Adolescent Psychiatry). If treatment is indicated, one place to start looking is through the government's treatment locator services (1-800-662-4357 or http://findtreatment.samhsa.org), which are supported by the Substance Abuse and Mental Health Services Administration in the U.S. Department of Health and Human Services. Substance use treatment is individualized and includes a comprehensive approach to address relevant factors contributing to or resulting from substance use. The setting for treatment is based on an assessment involving level of intoxication and potential for withdrawal; presence of other medical conditions; presence of other emotional, behavioral, or cognitive conditions; readiness or motivation to change; risk of relapse or continued drug use; and recovery environment (e.g., family, peers, school, legal system). Program settings include outpatient or intensive outpatient treatment, partial hospitalization, or residential or inpatient treatment. There are multiple evidence-based treatment approaches available, including those that use behavioral approaches, family-based approaches, addiction medications, and recovery support services (National Institute on Drug Abuse 2014).

Developmental Disabilities

In addition to school-based services, children with developmental disabilities may receive additional services through the community, whether funded privately or publicly. A *developmental disability* is defined by the Centers for Disease Control and Prevention as a condition "due to an impairment in physical, learning, language, or behavior areas. These conditions begin during the developmental period, may impact day-to-day functioning, and usually last throughout a person's lifetime" (Center for Disease Control and Prevention 2018).

States vary widely in how services for individuals with developmental disabilities are organized. In some states, services are provided by the same agencies that provide mental health services. In other states, services are under the same umbrella as other health-related services. In California, regional centers through the Department of Developmental Services provide local services such as assessment, diagnosis, counseling, lifelong individualized planning and services coordination, early intervention, family support, placement, and monitoring (https://dds.ca.gov). Some states contract out services to other providers. The National Association of State Directors of Developmental Disabilities Services is a good starting place to find appropriate state programs (www.nasddds.org/MemberAgencies/index.shtml). Conditions covered and eligibility for services vary from state to state. Developmental disabilities typically covered by states include intellectual disabilities and autism spectrum disorders.

Juvenile Justice and Probation

In 2013, an estimated 1,058,500 delinquency cases were handled by courts with juvenile jurisdiction (Hockenberry and Puzzanchera 2015). Even more cases are diverted out of the system prior to juvenile court intake. When a minor is charged with criminal behavior, he or she may be detained in a juvenile facility or may receive community supervision through probation. Juveniles in custody continue to receive educational services even while in a short- or long-term custodial setting. Juveniles out of custody may continue to attend their community school or may require a higher level of services in residential placement that involves on-site education services or coordination with a local off-site school.

When juveniles are supervised out of custody on probation, the minor's probation officer may coordinate with the school regarding the youth's needs, terms of probation, or whether his or her behavior at school is acceptable. Probation services, operated through state or local agencies depending on the particular state, are often the gateway to individual service needs (e.g., mental health treatment, substance use treatment, sexual offender treatment, family services) and require coordination with community agencies. For accessible resources and further information on juvenile justice, see the website of the Office of Juvenile Justice and Delinquency Prevention (www.ojjdp.gov).

Child Welfare System

As discussed in great depth in Chapter 4, "Danger at Home," children and adolescents can become involved with the child welfare system when child maltreatment occurs or is suspected. School officials are required to report suspected maltreatment to child protective services (CPS) when it comes to their attention. In addition to investigating and assessing maltreatment allegations, CPS may also provide services to the youth, again often including coordination with various community agencies. Services may be preventative or post-response. During 2016, approximately 1.3 million children received post-response services from a CPS agency. Services were provided to children and their families, both in their home and in foster care, in order to prevent future instances of child maltreatment and remedy conditions that brought the child and family to the attention of CPS (Children's Bureau 2018).

Preventative Interventions
Promoting Alternative Thinking Strategies

Promoting Alternative Thinking Strategies (PATHS) is a school-based social-emotional learning program designed to reduce aggression and other problematic behaviors in elementary school students, ranging from preschool through sixth grade. Additional information can be found at www.pathstraining.com/main.

LifeSkills Training

LifeSkills Training is a school-based program designed to prevent violence, drug use, and alcohol use among middle school–age youth. The program focuses on helping students increase self-esteem, improve coping skills, increase their knowledge about substance use, and gain helpful skills to resist peer pressure surrounding drug use. More information on this program can be found at www.lifeskillstraining.com.

Positive Action

Positive Action is a school-based program designed for elementary and middle school students that seeks to improve academic performance along with reducing substance use and violent behavior. Students are taught a series of 15- to 20-minute lessons throughout the year that have been shown to produce a variety of positive outcomes. Additional information about Positive Action can be found at www.positiveaction.net.

Gang Resistance and Education Training

Gang Resistance and Education Training (GREAT) is a school-, family-, and community-based program designed to reduce violence, prevent criminal behavior, and decrease the likelihood of gang involvement among youth. A randomized controlled trial of GREAT involving just over 3,800 ethnically diverse students from seven major cities across the United States found that participation in GREAT led to significantly improved attitudes toward police, established a less positive view of gangs, reduced risk-taking behaviors, and led to a 24% reduction in odds of gang membership 4 years out of the program (Esbensen et al. 2013). Interestingly, a recent meta-analysis based on six qualifying studies (Wong et al. 2016) looking at the effects of gang prevention programs on gang membership indicated that such programs may be beneficial. However, a closer look revealed that the positive benefits attributable to such programs are based entirely on the results of the study by Ebsensen and colleagues. This meta-analysis solidified GREAT as the only evidence-based prevention program. That said, the absence of many well-conducted studies on the effect of gang prevention programs does not mean that other gang prevention programs do not work. Rather, the meta-analysis referenced here underscores the need for more studies on the effect of gang prevention programs.

Family-Based Interventions

Psychosocial interventions that focus largely on the dynamics within a family are often the treatment of choice for youth who are prone to displays of violence. These interventions apply to youth from elementary school, to middle school, and on through high school. Some of these approaches, such as parent management training (PMT), primarily focus on working with parents. Others, such as functional family therapy (FFT) and brief strategic family therapy (BSFT), involve the whole family. For some teens involved with the juvenile justice system, multisystemic therapy (MST) is used. MST empowers parents to take the reins within the family and work closely with community resources (e.g., school, juvenile court, mental health professionals) in addressing criminal and violent behaviors.

Parent Management Training

PMT is a treatment approach based on social learning theory and is designed to address parenting practices associated with aggressive and oppositional behavior. One of PMT's core components involves helping parents build a more stable and secure relationship with their child through play. PMT also teaches parents how to provide incentives for their child to engage in prosocial behavior through rewards and healthy doses of positive reinforcement. Parents are also instructed on how to create well-defined house rules and consequences for misbehavior. Some particularly successful approaches that are based on a PMT model include The Incredible Years (www.incredibleyears.com), the Triple P Positive Parenting Program (https://www.triplep.net/glo-en/home), and parent-child interaction therapy. PMT is often the modality of first choice for preschool, elementary school, and middle school students.

Functional Family Therapy

FFT seeks to address the dysfunctional relationship patterns that exist within a family (Henggeler and Sheidow 2012). Some of the goals of FFT include improving communication between family members and increasing parental supervision. FFT is generally composed of three phases: the engagement and motivation phase, the behavior change phase, and the generalization phase. In the first phase, the therapist focuses on building a rapport with the family while focusing on the interpersonal relationship within the family rather than the child's problematic behavior. In the second phase, the family is guided in developing more constructive problem-solving-oriented approaches to address conflicts within the family. In the final phase, a focus is placed on helping the family apply the principles they have learned in a variety of contexts. FFT can be a particularly useful intervention for middle schoolers and high school students.

Brief Strategic Family Therapy

BSFT is an approach to family therapy that views a child's problematic behaviors as the products of a family system in distress. BSFT seeks to change the expectations and status quo within a family by modifying family member roles as well as addressing resistance to change. BSFT was originally developed for use with youth with a history of aggressive behavior and rule violations from Hispanic families in Miami, Florida. BSFT has since been shown to be effective for youth with a variety of ethnic backgrounds and behavior problems (Henggeler and Sheidow 2012). BFST is another approach that may be particularly useful in students from middle school through high school.

Multisystemic Therapy

MST was designed for youth who have serious behavior problems that have led to involvement with the juvenile justice system. MST addresses the factors that perpetuate serious behavior problems, including juvenile delinquency and substance abuse, at the individual, family, school, and community levels. MST involves a therapist who works with a family by going into the home, school, or other environments and is on call 24 hours a day. The therapist seeks to empower parents to take on a more active role in monitoring their child and to improve communication with other important players (e.g., school, juvenile court, mental health providers). The ultimate goal is for the therapist to hand off responsibility to the parents over time as the family's functioning improves. MST has been shown to lower re-arrest rates, improve families' psychosocial functioning, and reduce the likelihood that a child's younger siblings will become involved in the juvenile justice system (Henggeler 2012; Henggeler et al. 1992; van der Stouwe et al. 2014; Wagner et al. 2014). MST is not available in all counties across the United States; however, some counties use wraparound services that are akin to the approach taken in MST. MST is a particularly good option for middle schoolers and high school students who have committed violent acts and other criminal behaviors leading to juvenile justice system involvement.

Conclusion

The programs described in this chapter (Figure 10–2) are meant to familiarize mental health providers, school officials, and parents with the approaches currently employed to reduce school violence. However, there is much variability in regard to accessing community support, violence prevention programs, specialized mental health interventions, or even mental health providers. It is our hope that this summary will

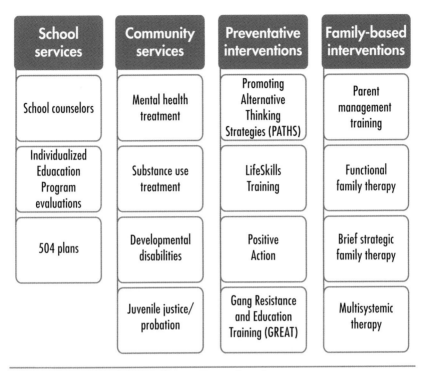

FIGURE 10–2. **Map of services in place.**

help schools and families use resources within their area and inspire the creation of more services for at-risk youth.

Case Vignette *(continued)*

When meeting with Lorraine, the counselor notes that her hair is somewhat messy and she has a stain on the sleeve of her blouse. Lorraine pauses a bit longer than expected before answering questions, and she occasionally scans the room. When asked about her story, Lorraine becomes visibly frustrated and says that it was "fictional" and that she does not "appreciate people bothering" her over the assignment. Lorraine is asked about her leisure activities and describes videos she has been watching on YouTube. Lorraine says she has learned a lot about the CIA's Project MK-ULTRA and mind-control drugs that are being surreptitiously administered to students around the country at school.

The counselor contacts Lorraine's mother, who shares that she works two jobs to support her daughter and Lorraine's uncle, an Iraq war veteran with debilitating posttraumatic stress disorder. Lorraine's mother states that her daughter has been keeping to herself more the past year, and she attributes this to Lorraine being a typical "moody teenager." When asked about Lorraine's access to weapons, she says that Lorraine's uncle keeps a semiautomatic rifle under his bed. After meeting with Lorraine and obtaining further information on risk factors for Lorraine, the counselor forms a plan for intervention (Table 10–2).

TABLE 10–2. Risk factors and intervention plan for Lorraine

Risk factor	Plan
Imminent danger to others	Refer Lorraine for psychiatric hospitalization. Inform law enforcement and school administration about potential danger (*Tarasoff* obligation; see Chapter 8, "Hostile Intent").
Mental health symptoms	Lorraine will require a psychiatric evaluation to determine a mental health diagnosis and treatment plan.
Possible access to weapons	Speak to Lorraine's mother about restricting access to weapons.
Academic decline	Once Lorraine is discharged, her mother should request Individualized Education Program evaluation to determine if Lorraine is eligible for special education services.
Ongoing violence risk	Lorraine should be closely monitored by a mental health team, who should routinely inquire about danger to others.

Key Points

- Primary, secondary, and tertiary interventions are available to prevent violence—with increasing numerical classification reflecting more narrowly defined target audience with greater risk of violence.

- Parent management training is a highly effective approach for addressing disruptive and violent behaviors in grade school and middle school children.

Clinical Pearls
School staff should be familiar with interventions that are available in the community and how students can access these services.
Getting buy-in from a student's caregivers (e.g., parents, foster parents) is essential for successfully implementing family-based interventions.

References

Americans With Disabilities Act of 1990, 42 USC §12101 (amended 2008)

Center for Disease Control and Prevention: Developmental disabilities: facts. Atlanta, GA, Center for Disease Control and Prevention, 2018. Available at: www.cdc.gov/ncbddd/developmentaldisabilities/facts.html. Accessed on March 28, 2019.

Children's Bureau: Child Maltreatment 2016. Washington, DC, Administration for Children and Families, U.S. Department of Health and Human Services, 2018. Available at: www.acf.hhs.gov/cb/resource/child-maltreatment-2016. Accessed April 16, 2019.

Esbensen F-A, Osgood DW, Peterson D, et al: Short- and long-term outcome results from a multisite evaluation of the GREAT program. Criminol Public Policy 12(3):375–411, 2013

Henggeler SW: Multisystemic therapy: clinical foundations and research outcomes. Psychosocial Intervention 21(2):181–193, 2012

Henggeler SW, Sheidow AJ: Empirically supported family based treatments for conduct disorder and delinquency in adolescents. J Marital Fam Ther 38(1):30–58, 2012 22283380

Henggeler SW, Melton GB, Smith LA: Family preservation using multisystemic therapy: an effective alternative to incarcerating serious juvenile offenders. J Consult Clin Psychol 60(6):953–961, 1992 1460157

Hockenberry S, Puzzanchera C: Juvenile Court Statistics 2013. Pittsburgh, PA, National Center for Juvenile Justice, 2015

Individuals with Disabilities Education Act, 20 U.S.C. § 1400 (2004)

National Institute on Drug Abuse: Principles of Adolescent Substance Use Disorder Treatment: A Research-Based Guide (Publ No 14-7953). Washington, DC, National Institutes of Health, 2014

Section 504 of the Rehabilitation Act of 1973, 29 USC § 794 (amended 2002)

van der Stouwe T, Asscher JJ, Stams GJJ, et al: The effectiveness of multisystemic therapy (MST): a meta-analysis. Clin Psychol Rev 34(6):468–481, 2014 25047448

Wagner DV, Borduin CM, Sawyer AM, et al: Long-term prevention of criminality in siblings of serious and violent juvenile offenders: a 25-year follow-up to a randomized clinical trial of multisystemic therapy. J Consult Clin Psychol 82(3):492–499, 2014 24417600

Wong JS, Gravel J, Bouchard M, et al: Promises kept? A meta-analysis of gang membership prevention programs. Journal of Criminological Research, Policy and Practice 2(2):134–147, 2016

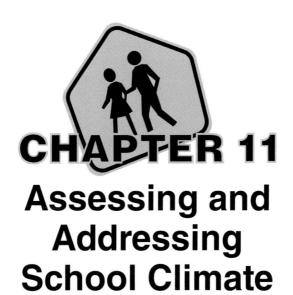

CHAPTER 11

Assessing and Addressing School Climate

Michael B. Kelly, M.D.

Anne B. McBride, M.D.

Jeff Bostic, M.D., Ed.D.

Sharon Hoover, Ph.D.

School isn't a waiting area for life.
It's where life happens for children. Every day.

Carol Jago

Perhaps the most important and impactful role a school system embodies in preventing violence is the duty of caring for the school environment. Consistent with the public health approach, schools fostering conditions that lead to safe and supportive learning environments are likely to promote positive behaviors among students and reduce the likelihood of negative outcomes, including school violence. Mechanisms to measure and improve school climate are increasingly gaining momentum, along with the evidence base that supports their usage. In this chapter, we provide guidance to school mental health clinicians on how to nurture fertile soil—how to assess and implement effective strategies that promote positive school climate.

According to the National Center on Safe Supportive Learning Environments (2011; NCSSLE), *school climate* can be conceptualized as how members of the school community experience interpersonal relationships, staff practices, and organizational structures. School climate includes the constructs of safety (both physical and emotional), connections and support among students and teachers and staff, and engagement of learners. Positive school climates reflect relationships that are respectful, trusting, and caring.

There is much evidence that learning environments with strong school climates promote a variety of positive outcomes for students, including both healthy social-emotional development and successful academic engagement (National Center on Safe Supportive Learning Environments 2011; Osher et al. 2008). Students in schools with positive learning environments that are safe, supportive, and engaging are more likely to improve academically and participate fully in the classroom and are less likely to exhibit disruptive classroom behaviors (MacNeil et al. 2009; Osher et al. 2008; Ripski and Gregory 2009). Furthermore, teachers who perceive their school to have a positive climate report lower levels of stress and burnout (Grayson and Alvarez 2008).

In recent years, the U.S. Department of Education (DOE) has prioritized efforts to help schools "create safer and more nurturing school climates." Newer federal legislation, the Every Student Succeeds Act (2015), encourages schools to consider assessing school climate as an indicator of overall school success. As such, many schools are looking for ways to measure school climate and identify interventions for improvement. In the following sections, we provide guidance on each of these areas as well as some general resources that may prove useful in efforts to improve school climate.

Measuring School Climate

To improve school climate, districts and schools must have reliable and valid mechanisms for assessment. A systematic process for collecting data from students, parents, and staff in a school or district offers a comprehensive perspective on how the school's important stakeholders perceive its climate. This sort of data collection enables data-driven decisions about preferred interventions and monitoring of progress. Although many assessments are available, the DOE recently developed an adaptable suite of surveys and an associated Web-based platform called the U.S. Department of Education School Climate Surveys (EDSCLS). The platform, available to schools, districts, and states, can be downloaded free of charge from the NCSSLE. The EDSCLS provides user-friendly school climate reports back to users in real time. The DOE also provides a manual, *Guiding Principles: A Resource Guide for Improving School Climate and Discipline* (U.S. Department of Education 2014), that is accessible online and addresses foundational principles on this topic.

The Authoritative School Climate Survey (ASCS; Cornell 2015) is accessible online and applicable for secondary students in grades 6–12 and elementary students in grades 3–5. Both student and teacher/staff versions of the ASCS are available at https://curry.virginia.edu/uploads/resourceLibrary/Authoritative_School_Climate_Survey_Research_Summary_1-31-16.pdf. Originally named the Virginia Secondary School Climate Survey, the ASCS is based on the authoritative school climate theory, which posits that "both structure and support are needed in order to maintain a safe and orderly school climate conducive to learning" (Cornell 2015, p. 2). The report clarifies, "Support is conceptualized as warmth and acceptance by teachers and staff whereas structure is defined as strict but fair enforcement of school rules and high academic expectations for students" (Cornell 2015, p. 2). The 2015 report summarizes the research supporting the authoritative school climate model and provides surveys for school climate and bullying assessments. Secondary surveys can generally be administered in 20–25 minutes, and the elementary version is even shorter.

Addressing School Climate

Multimodality tends to be a common thread woven through successful programs for preventing violence and treating underlying problems. That is, successful approaches for addressing violence generally involve some combination of interventions at the individual, family, school, and community levels. For instance, if the violent behavior of a student were the product of problems inherent to that student alone, then individual psychotherapy, and possibly medications in the case of reactive, affective, defensive, and impulsive (RADI) aggression, would solve most problems. However, the literature on youth violence, particularly in the areas of juvenile delinquency, disruptive behavior disorders, and violence risk assessment, shows us that violence is a complex tapestry of multilayered and dynamic processes (Steiner et al. 2017). Thus, the approaches we use to address violence in our schools must be dynamic and multilayered as well. In this chapter, we broadly describe the components of school-based programs that are designed to improve school climate as a means of preventing school violence and other problems. We also provide resources that teachers and school administrators can use to find a variety of structured interventions for improving school climate.

Approaches to Changing School Climate

In their report, a product of the School Discipline Consensus Project, a component of the Supportive School Discipline Initiative of the U.S. Departments of Education and Justice, Morgan et al. (2014) provided a valuable resource for school administrators that summarizes types of interventions that are used to improve school climate. Some of these interventions focus on helping curb disruptive behavior and improving relationships with peers (e.g., character education, social-emotional learning [SEL], positive youth development [PYD]). Another set of interventions currently being used in schools targets fostering an inclusive school community and responsiveness to students who are having difficulties (e.g., positive behavioral interventions and support [PBIS], restorative practices, School Development Program [SDP]).

Character Education

Character education programs focus on teaching developmentally appropriate social skills, instilling moral values, and reducing bullying behavior. The principles of character education programs have long been applied in schools with a religious affiliation. Character education programs have also been a source of controversy. For example, some people have argued that character education programs are a one-size-fits-all approach that conflates conforming to behavioral norms with moral development (Kohn 1997; Whitley 2007). Furthermore, studies looking at the effectiveness of character education programs have not yielded data suggesting that they have a discernible impact on students' moral values, social skills, and other behaviors (Social and Character Development Research Consortium 2010). Despite the lack of evidence for such programs, we acknowledge that the decision on whether to use a character education program in schools is ultimately up to the school's administration, parents, and the community.

Social-Emotional Learning

SEL programs focus on helping students improve skills related to recognizing and dealing with emotions, increasing empathy for peers, and improving their relationships. Such programs value bolstering "EQ over IQ" in preparing students for the adult world. That is, SEL approaches seek to improve students' emotional literacy in order to reduce campus violence, improve cohesiveness among the student body, and teach the importance of grit when pursuing goals. *Grit* is a neurocognitive trait defined by Duckworth et al. (2007, p. 1087) as "perseverance and passion for long-term goals" that has been shown to be a predictive measure for future success. In fact, some studies suggest that the persistent effort and application of talent in the face of adversity that characterizes grit has a larger influence on success in life than does intelligence (Abuhassàn and Bates 2015; Duckworth et al. 2007). Grit can be an important focus for improvement among students with SEL challenges.

A meta-analysis by Durlak et al. (2011) based on data from more than 270,000 students compared schools with and without SEL programs. The meta-analysis revealed that SEL program participation was associated with reductions in school violence and disruptive behavior as well as improved academic performance. Thus, SEL appears to be an effective primary prevention strategy for reducing school violence.

Positive Youth Development

PYD, like the SEL approach just described, has a solid foundation of evidence behind it. PYD programs use strength-based approaches to introduce or enhance the protective factors associated with keeping youth on track developmentally. Activities associated with PYD include participation in youth sports, after-school programs, groups focused on exploring cultural identity, and 4-H. There is evidence that PYD approaches have been associated with improved academic performance and reductions in antisocial behavior (Fredricks and Simpkins 2012). Thus, PYD programs show promise as secondary prevention for school violence.

Positive Behavioral Interventions and Support

PBIS is a primary, secondary, and tertiary prevention program designed to reduce school violence, promote academic success, and improve school climate. PBIS approaches involve establishing clear and consistent expectations for classroom behavior and consequences for disruptive behavior. Rather than suspension or removing students from class, the PBIS model tries to keep students in the classroom and reinforce prosocial behaviors. The current literature indicates that PBIS approaches are associated with improved school climate and reduced bullying. However, more studies are needed in order to make more conclusive recommendations (Bradshaw 2015).

Restorative Practices

School-based restorative practice programs focus on teaching students conflict resolution skills that are put into action when transgressions occur. This approach stems from criminal and juvenile justice literature that details restorative justice approaches. In these approaches, perpetrators meet with victims in order to take personal accountability for their actions and come to an agreement on how to make amends. A review by Fronius et al. (2016) pointed out that a limited amount of data suggests that restorative practices in schools are helpful in improving school climate; however, the evidence base for this approach is still in its infancy.

School Development Program

The SDP was developed in the late 1960s at the Yale Child Study Center in order to address educational disparities for low-income youth from ethnic minority backgrounds. This approach uses different teams that focus on school planning and management; student and staff support; and parents and families, whose input is used in making a comprehensive plan. Schools that undergo the SDP process have demonstrated positive changes in school climate marked by improved academic performance and increases in prosocial behavior (Lunenburg 2011).

Trauma-Informed Approach

Before concluding our discussion of school-based interventions to improve school climate, we wish to underscore the importance of a trauma-informed approach. According to the U.S. Department of Health and Human Services (Children's Bureau 2012), the rate of child victimization in 2012 alone was 8.7 per 1,000 children in boys and 9.5 per 1,000 children in girls. Given the ubiquity of trauma, a trauma-informed approach to mental health interventions at school is essential. The Substance Abuse and Mental Health Services Administration (2017) characterizes trauma-informed programs (e.g., school-based mental health services) as having the following characteristics:

1. Realizes the widespread impact of trauma and understands potential paths to recovery
2. Recognizes the signs and symptoms of trauma in youth, families, staff, and others involved with the system
3. Responds by fully integrating knowledge about trauma into policies, procedures, and practices
4. Seeks to actively resist retraumatization

It is important that both the programs being implemented and the people implementing them (e.g., school administrators, teachers, school nurses, mental health providers) receive proper training in this area and keep these principles in mind when working with students. For a more comprehensive summary regarding a trauma-informed approach to addressing school violence, see Chapter 4, "Danger at Home."

TABLE 11–1. **Guides for improving school climate**

Resource	Description
Quick Guide for Making School Climate Improvements (https://safesupportive learning.ed.gov/scirp/quick-guide)	This helpful guide summarizes basic information on how to go about improving school climate.
Reference Manual on Making School Climate Improvements (https://safe supportivelearning.ed.gov/scirp/ reference-manual)	This manual includes a summary of goals, strategies, and resources for going about improving school climate.

Conclusion

Interventions that improve school climate are a commonsense way of reducing the likelihood of school violence. It is our hope that the resources in this chapter offer a path forward for school districts that are grappling with the complex problem of school violence. Web links to some helpful online resources for improving school climate are provided in Table 11–1.

Key Points

- Learning environments with strong school climates promote a variety of positive outcomes for students, including both healthy social-emotional development and successful academic engagement.

- Successful approaches for addressing violence generally involve some combination of interventions at the individual, family, school, and community levels.

Clinical Pearl

The EDSCLS to assess school climate can be downloaded free of charge from the NCSSLE website at https://safesupportivelearning.ed.gov/edscls.

References

Abuhassàn A, Bates TC: Grit: distinguishing effortful persistence from consci-
entiousness. J Individ Differ 36:205–214, 2015

Bradshaw CP: Translating research to practice in bullying prevention. Am Psychol 70(4):322–332, 2015 25961313

Children's Bureau: Child Maltreatment 2012. Washington, DC, Administration
for Children and Families, U.S. Department of Health and Human Services,
2012. Available from www.acf.hhs.gov/sites/default/files/cb/cm2012.pdf.
Accessed March 29, 2019.

Cornell D: The Authoritative School Climate Survey and the School Climate Bullying Survey: Research Summary. Charlottesville, VA, Curry School of Education, University of Virginia. 2015. Available at: http://curry.virginia.edu/
uploads/resourceLibrary/Authoritative_School_Climate_Survey_Research_
Summary_1-31-16.pdf. Accessed March 29, 2019.

Duckworth AL, Peterson C, Matthews MD, et al: Grit: perseverance and passion
for long-term goals. J Pers Soc Psychol 92(6):1087–1101, 2007 17547490

Durlak JA, Weissberg RP, Dymnicki AB, et al: The impact of enhancing students'
social and emotional learning: a meta-analysis of school-based universal interventions. Child Dev 82(1)405–432, 2011 21291449

Every Student Succeeds Act, Pub.L. 114-95, 2015

Fredricks JA, Simpkins SD: Promoting positive youth development through organized after-school activities: taking a closer look at participation of ethnic
minority youth. Child Dev Perspect 6(3):280–287, 2012

Fronius T, Persson H, Guckenburg S, et al: Restorative Justice in U.S. Schools: A
Research Review. San Francisco, CA, WestEd Justice and Prevention Training Center, 2016

Grayson JL, Alvarez HK: School climate factors relating to teacher burnout: a
mediator model. Teaching and Teacher Education 24(5):1349–1363, 2008

Kohn A: How not to teach values: a critical look at character education. Phi
Delta Kappan 78(6):429–439, 1997

Lunenburg FC: The Comer School Development Program: improving education
for low-income students. National Forum of Multicultural Issues Journal
8(1):1–14, 2011

MacNeil AJ, Prater DL, Busch S: The effects of school culture and climate on student
achievement. International Journal of Leadership in Education 12(1):73–84,
2009

Morgan E, Salomon N, Plotkin M, et al: The School Discipline Consensus Report:
Strategies From the Field to Keep Students Engaged in School and Out of the
Juvenile Justice System. New York, Council of State Governments Justice
Center, 2014

National Center on Safe Supportive Learning Environments: Making the Case
for the Importance of School Climate and Its Measurement (webinar).
Washington, DC, National Center on Safe Supportive Learning Environments, 2011. Available at: http://safesupportivelearning.ed.gov/events/
webinar/making-case-importance-school-climate-and-its-measurement.
Accessed March 29, 2019.

Osher D, Kendziora K, Chinen M: Student Connection Research: Final Narrative Report to the Spencer Foundation. Washington, DC, American Institutes for Research, 2008. Available at: www.air.org/resource/student-connection-research-final-narrative-report-spencer-foundation. Accessed March 29, 2019.

Ripski MB, Gregory A: Unfair, unsafe, and unwelcome: do high school students' perceptions of unfairness, hostility, and victimization in school predict engagement and achievement? J Sch Violence 8(4):355–375, 2009

Social and Character Development Research Consortium: Efficacy of Schoolwide Programs to Promote Social and Character Development and Reduce Problem Behavior in Elementary School Children. Washington, DC, National Center for Education Research, Institute of Education Sciences, U.S. Department of Education, 2010

Steiner H, Daniels W, Stadler C, et al: Disruptive Behavior: Development, Psychopathology, Crime, and Treatment. New York, Oxford University Press, 2017.

Substance Abuse and Mental Health Services Administration: Trauma-Informed Approach and Trauma-Specific Interventions. Rockville, MD, National Center for Trauma-Informed Care and Alternatives to Seclusion and Restraint, Substance Abuse and Mental Health Services Administration, 2017. Available at: www.samhsa.gov/nctic/trauma-interventions. Accessed September 20, 2017.

U.S. Department of Education: Guiding Principles: A Resource Guide for Improving School Climate and Discipline. Washington, DC, U.S. Department of Education, 2014. Available at: www2.ed.gov/policy/gen/guid/school-discipline/guiding-principles.pdf. Accessed March 29, 2019.

Whitley JG: Reversing the Perceived Moral Decline in American Schools: A Critical Literature Review of America's Attempt at Character Education. Williamsburg, VA, College of William and Mary, 2007

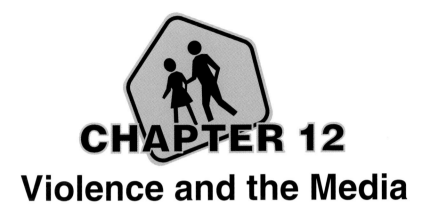

CHAPTER 12
Violence and the Media

Michael B. Kelly, M.D.

Suzanne Shimoyama, M.D.

*One need only posit some threat to the public tranquility and
any action can be justified.*

Leo Tolstoy

Case Vignette

Mark is a 15-year-old sophomore. Although he had a few friends in elementary school, he has always struggled socially. Now that he is in high school, he has the reputation of being a "loner." Mark's teachers describe him as an average to below-average student and say that he is polite but tends to keep to himself. Recently, Mark was targeted by a small group of classmates, who began bullying him. It started with verbal insults that humiliated Mark in front of his peers but later escalated to deliberate pushing and bumping in the halls and threats of greater violence. After several weeks of enduring the bullying without retaliation, Mark "snapped." He advised the bullies that he was armed and warned that if they touched him again, they would regret it. A female student overheard the exchange and informed school staff, who detained Mark and searched his backpack and locker. In his locker they found two large hunting knives.

After discovering the weapons in Mark's locker, staff notified school police and called in Mark's parents. Mark's parents expressed that they were shocked by what happened, stating that Mark had never been in trouble at school before and did not have behavioral problems at home. They explained that they both worked long hours and that Mark spent most of his time home alone in his room on his computer playing video games. His parents were not aware of the content of these games because they never felt there was a need to closely supervise him, although they did express concern regarding his lack of friends and apparent lack of interest in socializing. After an investigation, police found that Mark spent up to 8 hours a day playing violent video games, mostly first-person shooters. They also found that he had made a vague allusion to planning to "take revenge" on his tormentors on a video game message board.

Following an act of violence, particularly one that is perpetrated by a child or adolescent, it is common for people to want answers. They ask, "How could this have happened?" "Why did he do it?" "Who could have prevented this?" Shortly thereafter, blame is ascribed: "It's the parents' fault." "The mental health system should have identified him as a risk." "His peers should have been nicer to him." In the past few decades, the target of blame has shifted to the media. After the Columbine shooting in 1999, politicians, reporters, and pundits blamed the shooting on the teenage killers' fandom of shock rocker Marilyn Manson, their affinity for the first-person shooter video game Doom, and supposed identification with characters from the film *The Matrix*. President Bill Clinton ordered an investigation into the marketing of violent entertainment, and the victims' families filed a lawsuit against 25 video game makers, seeking $5 billion in damages. Following the Sandy Hook shooting in 2012, media sources began linking the event to the killer's interest in video games. Most recently, after the Parkland school shooting in 2018, the debate over the role of violent media once again took center stage, with President Donald Trump stating, "I'm hearing more and more people say the level of violence on video games is really shaping young people's thoughts" (Ducharme 2018).

Violent Media

Researchers have long sought to understand what role, if any, exposure to violent media plays in acts of violence committed by young people. In the early 1960s, the classic Bobo doll experiments by Bandura et al. (1963) contributed to their social learning theory. These experiments demonstrated that children who were exposed to an aggressive model, whether it was a live person, a person on film, or a cartoon, were more likely to exhibit aggressive behavior following the exposure than children who were not exposed to an aggressive model. This concept of imitable violence has contributed significantly to network television broadcast standards and practices. Following the Columbine mass shooting in 1999, Fox Family Worldwide made significant changes to their guidelines for fantasy violence and action shows such as the popular children's program *Mighty Morphin Power Rangers* in an attempt to reduce the potential for imitable violent behavior by its viewers. Some of these guidelines included the nonrealistic portrayal of weapons that would shoot lasers rather than bullets (Bryant 2014).

Organizations such as the American Academy of Pediatrics (AAP) and American Academy of Child and Adolescent Psychiatry (AACAP) have issued policy statements drawing links between media violence and behavior. In 2009 the AAP described the impact of exposure to violence through various media outlets (e.g., television, video games, music) and concluded that exposure to media violence is associated with desensitization to violence, generation of anxiety related to being victimized, and an increase in physical aggression (Council on Communications and Media 2009). Recent neuroimaging data appear to substantiate the AAP's concerns: areas of the prefrontal cortex responsible for regulating emotions and behavior are altered in response to exposure to violent media (Hummer 2015).

Several additional studies support the AAP's stance. A meta-analysis by Anderson et al. (2010) involving youth from Western countries and Japan showed that exposure to violent video games was associated with reduced empathy. Such exposure was shown to be a risk factor for aggressive thinking, emotions, and behavior regardless of gender or cultural background. Another large meta-analysis (Greitemeyer and Mügge 2014) with data from 98 studies and nearly 37,000 participants found that violent video games were associated with aggression and reductions in prosocial behavior; however, games with prosocial themes were shown to have a positive impact. Additional studies have found that playing video games with prosocial themes increased empathy in individuals who played them (Greitemeyer et al. 2010; Prot et al. 2014).

People who disagree that violent media plays a central role in violent behavior argue that violent media exists all over the world, yet countries such as Japan, Australia, and South Korea do not experience violence at the same level as the United States (Fisher 2012; United Nations Office on Drugs and Crime 2013). They also point out that the vast majority of youth who play violent video games do not commit violent acts. In the landmark case Brown v. Entertainment Merchants Association (2011), in a 7–2 decision, the Supreme Court struck down a California law banning the sale of violent video games to children. In the decision, Justice Antonin Scalia wrote, "Psychological studies purporting to show a connection between exposure to violent video games and harmful effects on children do not prove that such exposure causes minors to act aggressively. Any demonstrated effects are both small and indistinguishable from effects produced by other media."

Some research has not supported the notion that exposure to media violence is associated with real world violent acts. For example, a study by Ferguson et al. (2012) and a meta-analysis by Ferguson (2015) indicated that violent video games are not associated with aggression. In his

2015 meta-analysis, Ferguson held publication bias (i.e., the selective publishing of studies with positive results) potentially responsible for some previous studies portraying violent video games as having negative effects on youth. A particularly interesting study by Szycik et al. (2017) sought to answer the question of whether long-term exposure to violent video games blunts our brain's responses to emotionally charged stimuli. Longtime enthusiasts of violent video games and control subjects were hooked up to a functional magnetic resonance imaging brain scanner and were shown pictures meant to evoke a range of emotional responses. Much to the delight of middle schoolers everywhere, neither violent video game players nor control subjects showed evidence that their neural responses to emotionally charged stimuli had been blunted.

A recent meta-analysis by Prescott et al. (2018) attempted to address several of Ferguson's criticisms. After assessing for publication bias and including adequate statistical controls, the authors concluded that "playing violent video games is associated with greater levels of overt physical aggression over time, after accounting for prior aggression" (Prescott et al. 2018, p. 6). Consistent with these findings, many experts, including the AACAP, suggest that parents limit their children's exposure to violent media (e.g., violent video games, movies, television). Although we agree with the AACAP's recommendation that caregivers limit children's exposure to violent media, it is important to note that the association between media violence (e.g., violent video games) and aggression does not imply causation. On the basis of the current literature, generalizations suggesting that violent video games cause violent behavior are a gross oversimplification.

Case Vignette *(continued)*

On further investigation, police found in Mark's Internet browser history links to news stories about recent school shootings as well as inquiries into the identities of the killers. Transcripts from Mark's online chats revealed statements he made about famous massacres that indicated an admiration for the killers. During the police investigation, Mark was also evaluated by a mental health professional. Mark reported that he had not always harbored violent fantasies but over the past few years felt an increasing sense of isolation and loneliness. He described his video games as an "escape" where he could feel powerful and effective. He said that he could relate to school shooters he read about in that they appeared to be social outcasts as well. When asked if he had planned to act on any of his violent fantasies, he responded, "I don't know."

Role of the Media

The role the media plays in real-world violence extends beyond the content of violent television, movies, and video games. The news media's coverage of violence in schools appears to have other effects as well. For example, following the release of footage of a school shooting in Colorado, a Gallup poll revealed that two-thirds of Americans reported they believed a similar event could occur in their own community school (Saad 1999 as cited in Cornell 2009). However, according to a simple calculation by Cornell obtained by dividing the number of American schools (~120,000) by the number of school shootings (103 between 1992–1993 and 2003–2004), each school would be expected to have a shooting approximately every 13,870 years (Cornell 2009). These data suggest that media coverage raises the American public's fears that they will be the unlikely victim of tragedy.

In addition, the media may play a role in inciting violence through contagion and copycat effects. A study by Towers et al. (2015) described the *apparent contagion effect* that is attributable to media coverage of mass shootings, including school shootings. That is, there is an observed increase in the likelihood of school shootings and similar gun-related crimes for approximately 13 days after a shooting event occurs. The authors also found an association between the degree of gun ownership within a state and the likelihood of mass shootings. Despite limited data on mass shootings, recent data appear to support the initial claims made by Towers and colleagues (Gould and Olivares 2017). In a recent paper, Meindl and Ivy (2017) proposed that the term *generalized imitation* does a better job of conveying the copycat nature of many mass shootings.

Many mass shooters crave the attention associated with their acts (Lankford 2016). For example, a recent article by Lankford and Madfis (2017) described how the Sandy Hook School shooter debated in online chat forums as to which was "the most famous school shooting." The authors suggested the following four guidelines for news media outlets in order to mitigate contagion and copycat effects:

1. Do not name the perpetrator.
2. Do not use photos or likenesses of the perpetrator.
3. Stop using the names, photos, or likenesses of past perpetrators.
4. Report everything else about these crimes in as much detail as desired.

The data reported by the various studies raise some important ethical questions for parents, educators, and media professionals. At what point does our freedom of speech encroach on the development of our youth? Do we need stricter laws governing what our children are exposed to in the media? Can media outlets be trusted to act with their communities' best interests in mind with regard to the type and timing of information they share, especially on the heels of mass shootings? It is beyond the scope of this book to answer such questions; however, the authors advocate for a commonsense approach to discussing mass shootings in the media, as proposed by Lankford and Madfis (2017). We also agree with the AAP and AACAP recommendations that parents limit and monitor young people's exposure to violence in the media.

Key Points

- Recent meta-analyses have shown associations between violent video game play and aggression; however, a causal relationship has not been established.

- The concept of imitable violence (i.e., violence that can be readily imitated) has influenced guidelines for broadcast standards and practices of programming targeting children.

- Although exposure to media violence has not been proven to cause violent behavior, we recommend that parents set limits on and monitor their children's exposure to violent media.

- Research suggests that refraining from naming and sharing additional details about perpetrators of mass shootings may detract from the infamy that attracts some school shooters to commit such violence.

Clinical Pearls

Although violent video game play appears to be associated with increased aggression, currently, there is no conclusive evidence that playing violent video games increases the likelihood that a student will become violent at school.

Clinicians are advised to recommend that caretakers limit and monitor their children's access to violent media content.

References

Council on Communications and Media: From the American Academy of Pediatrics: policy statement—media violence. Pediatrics 124(5):1495–1503, 2009 19841118

Anderson CA, Shibuya A, Ihori N, et al: Violent video game effects on aggression, empathy, and prosocial behavior in Eastern and Western countries: a meta-analytic review. Psychol Bull 136(2):151–173, 2010 20192553

Bandura A, Ross D, Ross SA: Imitation of film-mediated aggressive models. J Abnorm Soc Psychol 66(1):3–11, 1963 13966304

Brown v. Entertainment Merchants Association, 131 S. Ct. 2729, 564 U.S. 786, 180 L. Ed. 2d 708 (2011).

Bryant JA (ed): The Children's Television Community. New York, Routledge, 2014

Cornell DG: The Virginia Model for Student Threat Assessment. Workshop at the XIV Workshop Aggression. Berlin, Germany, Freie Universitat, November 2009

Ducharme J: Trump blames video games for school shootings: here's what science says. Time, March 8, 2018. Available at: www.time.com/5191182/trump-video-games-violence. Accessed March 24, 2019.

Ferguson CJ: Do Angry Birds make for angry children? A meta-analysis of video game influences on children's and adolescents' aggression, mental health, prosocial behavior, and academic performance. Perspect Psychol Sci 10(5):646–666, 2015 26386002

Ferguson CJ, San Miguel C, Garza A, et al: A longitudinal test of video game violence influences on dating and aggression: a 3-year longitudinal study of adolescents. J Psychiatr Res 46(2):141–146, 2012 22099867

Fisher M: Ten-country comparison suggests there's little or no link between video games and gun murders. The Washington Post, December 17, 2012

Gould MS, Olivares M: Mass shootings and murder-suicide: review of the empirical evidence for contagion, in Media and Suicide: International Perspectives on Research, Theory, and Policy. New York, Routledge, 2017, pp 41–66

Greitemeyer T, Mügge DO: Video games do affect social outcomes: a meta-analytic review of the effects of violent and prosocial video game play. Pers Soc Psychol Bull 40(5):578–589, 2014 24458215

Greitemeyer T, Osswald S, Brauer M: Playing prosocial video games increases empathy and decreases schadenfreude. Emotion 10(6):796–802, 2010 21171755

Hummer TA: Media violence effects on brain development: what neuroimaging has revealed and what lies ahead. Am Behav Sci 59(14):1790–1806, 2015

Lankford A: Fame seeking-rampage shooters: initial findings and empirical predictions. Aggress Violent Behav 27:122–129, 2016

Lankford A, Madfis E: Don't name them, don't show them, but report everything else: a pragmatic proposal for denying mass killers the attention they seek and deterring future offenders. Am Behav Sci 62(2):260–279, 2017

Meindl JN, Ivy JW: Mass shootings: the role of the media in promoting generalized imitation. Am J Public Health 107(3):368–370, 2017 28103074

Prescott AT, Sargent JD, Hull JG: Metaanalysis of the relationship between violent video game play and physical aggression over time. Proc Natl Acad Sci USA 115(40):9882–9888, 2018 30275306

Prot S, Gentile DA, Anderson CA, et al: Long-term relations among prosocial-media use, empathy, and prosocial behavior. Psychol Sci 25(2):358–368, 2014 24335350

Saad L: Public views Littleton tragedy as sign of deeper problems in country. Gallup News Service, April 23, 1999

Szycik GR, Mohammadi B, Münte TF, et al: Lack of evidence that neural empathic responses are blunted in excessive users of violent video games: an fMRI study. Front Psychol 8:174, 2017 28337156

Towers S, Gomez-Lievano A, Khan M, et al: Contagion in mass killings and school shootings. PLoS One 10(7):e0117259, 2015 26135941

United Nations Office on Drugs and Crime: Global Study on Homicide 2013 (Sales No 14.IV.1). Vienna, Austria, United Nations Office on Drugs and Crime, 2013

Afterword

Despite some recent high-profile tragedies, American schools in general are among the safest they have ever been (Cornell 2017). However, violence in our schools remains an all too common phenomenon. Furthermore, access to quality education and exposure to violence vary greatly across our nation in regard to geography, socioeconomic status, and ethnicity. Therefore, blanket statements about the safety of our schools lack nuance and context. Similarly, approaches to addressing the threat and the risk of violence that a particular student or group of students in a school pose is highly dependent on the biological, psychological, and social factors that impact day-to-day life.

Recently, a 10-year-old boy who was interviewed in a psychiatric crisis setting was asked if he felt safe at school. He had disclosed that he was bullied at school, and the question seemed relevant. His answer was surprising. He said, "Last week a student walked into their school and killed 17 people. No, I don't feel safe at school." As child and adolescent forensic psychiatrists, we have encountered similar storylines numerous times.

The following week, a 13-year-old boy was brought to the crisis center in handcuffs by three law enforcement officers after concern was raised about an inappropriate comment he made about a bomb. Although the youth voiced no intent to harm anyone, he was preoccupied with violent footage easily accessed through social media sites. He described participating in a mandatory school drill to practice the student body's response to a potential school shooter. He considered fearfully how easy it would have been for someone to kill people en masse after everyone had been herded into one auditorium.

These examples are not uncommon. As forensic evaluators, we have evaluated numerous youth who have been exposed to extreme levels of violence at home, in their communities, and, perhaps most unexpected and regrettably, at school. In our view, it is easy to get carried away focusing on the anger, horror, and fear that spring from violent tragedies in our schools. In reality, far too many youth grow up in communities or homes where violence is unavoidable. In general, children do not get to choose the environments where they are raised. In addition to environment, youth violence often involves a complex network of various factors such as temperament, developmental maturity, policy, culture, family, and biology, to name a few. Understanding the factors involved in the perpetration of violence is incredibly important both when healing from tragic events and in preventing future tragedies.

Youth can be remarkably resilient, apt to show substantial strength in the face of sometimes extreme adversity. In an ideal scenario, early identification affords the time to build on inherent resiliency and create the scaffolding for a healthier developmental trajectory. Schools often stand at the forefront of identifying at-risk youth early. Within the school setting, teachers, parents, school administrators, and mental health clinicians must make good use of opportusnities to work collaboratively in identifying children's individual needs and implementing interventions to strengthen our youth. Sometimes a relatively minor intervention can significantly alter a child's trajectory. In sum, focusing on the resiliency, malleability, and potential of youth is our best bet and a hopeful strategy for change.

Michael B. Kelly, M.D.
Anne B. McBride, M.D.

Reference

Cornell DG: School Violence: Fears Versus Facts. New York, Routledge, 2017

Appendix A

Example Threat Assessment Questions for Use With Grade School Students

Introduction to the Student

Introduce yourself, being sure to tell the student your name and role (e.g., school counselor, vice principal), and describe the purpose of the meeting (e.g., "I want to understand what happened today and figure out how to help"). Let the student know that you are working as part of a team and that the information you discuss will be shared with its members and parents and that he or she will not be forced to answer questions. Also, let the student know that he or she can tell you if there are fears related to sharing certain types of information so that you can think together about how those fears can be addressed (e.g., "It is okay if you ever feel too scared to tell me something. If that happens, we can talk about what you are worried about and how to help you feel safe.").

Initial Questions Regarding the Threat Incident

1. "Can you tell/show me what happened and when?"
2. "Did you say anything to/about [*target*]? What was said?"
3. "What did you mean when you said/did that?"
4. "How did you feel when that happened or when that was said?"
5. "How do you feel now?"
6. "How do you think [*target*] is/was feeling about what you said or did?"
7. "What do you want to do now?"

If the student resists talking about the incident, the clinician may employ more indirect questions such as the following:

1. "Tell me about your class/teacher this year." [*Notice whether the student has a negative or deteriorating perception of school this year.*]
2. "How do you like recess? What do you usually do?" [*Notice what the student is doing during less supervised time at school, potential bullying experiences, retreating from others, feeling excluded by peers, etc.*]
3. "Who do you like at this school? Do you have friends you ride the bus with? Who do you usually eat with?" [*Notice the student's connections with peers at school and if peers remain friends after the school day.*]
4. "What do you do when you leave school? What do you usually do after dinner?" [*Notice how the student's life is currently going outside school.*]
5. "What do like to do for fun? Who do you enjoy being with? Who in this school do you like to be around?"

Precipitants to Event

1. "What happened right before [*the incident*]?"
2. "Did something happen that made you say/do that?"
3. "Has anything else been bothering you?"
4. "Have you been feeling different? Has anything been making you upset? Or mad?"

Physical Evidence

1. "Did you get anything so that you could actually hurt/stab/shoot [*target*]?"
2. "Did you write/tell anyone about this?"
3. "Do you have a [*weapon*]? Where is it? Have you ever used it?" [*Notice whether the student expresses aggression toward animals or people.*]

Motives for Behavior

1. "Do you know why you did [*behavior*]?
2. "Do you know why [*that incident*] happened?"
3. "What did you wish would happen when you said/did [*incident*]?"
4. "Was there anything about [*target*] that made you do [*incident*]?"

Plan

1. "How long have you been thinking about doing [*threat*]?"
2. "Did you have to do anything to get ready to do [*threat*]?"

3. "Did you wait for a certain time or place to do [*threat*]?"
4. "Did you make plans for how to do [*threat*]?"

Accomplices

1. "Did you tell anyone about [*threat*]? Was there anyone you talked to about this?"
2. "Did anyone give you ideas about what to do?"
3. "Did anyone hear or know about this?"
4. "Did anyone try to stop you from doing this?"
5. "Did anyone help you?"

Target(s)

1. "What happened that made you say/do this to [*target*]?"
2. "Did you know you were going to say/do this to [*target*]?" [*Notice whether a particular person mattered.*]
3. "Is there anyone else you have felt this way about? Is there anyone you have felt like saying/doing this to?"
4. "Is there something that [*target*] does that makes you feel this way?"
5. "Do you still feel this way about [*target*]?"

Weapons

1. "Does anyone you live with keep a gun?"
2. "Have you ever used a [*knife, gun, rock, etc.*] before? What happened? How was that for you?"
3. "Can you get a [*weapon*] today if you needed one?"
4. "Have you ever used a [*weapon*] to protect yourself or hurt anyone?"

Detail Specificity and Plausibility

1. "What did you think would happen?"
2. "Did you have to change your plan because something happened or didn't work?"
3. "Did you have other ideas about how to get back at/harm [*target*]?"

Emotional Intensity

1. "Were you mad or upset when you said/did [*threat*]?"
2. "Do you remember what you said/did to [*target*]?"
3. "Have you felt this upset before? What else makes you this upset?"

Appendix B

Example Threat Assessment Questions for Use With Middle School Students

Introduction to the Student

Introduce yourself by name and clarify your role (e.g., school counselor, vice principal). Tell the student that you believe that his or her perspective on what happened is important and that you want to understand what happened. Tell the student that you may talk to others (e.g., target, witnesses, parents, teachers) and that he or she will not be forced to tell you anything. Tell the student that he or she can let you know if there is anything he or she feels afraid to discuss, and if so, you will work together on a solution.

If the adolescent shuts down or resists engaging, the clinician can take several steps to increase rapport with the student to elicit more complete information.

1. "This is a tough situation, and I can see you are between a rock and a hard place. I understand that you may not want to talk about this at all. But something made this happen, and I don't want to jump to any conclusions. I want your perspective on this."
2. "It sounds like things have been building up for a while with no way to fix it. Did you feel like something needed to happen? Can you help me understand what led up to this?"
3. Threats of calling the police if the student will not cooperate usually just intensify resistance. When more "power," particularly an unfamiliar other, is brought in, the student may feel more threatened and thus less safe to answer questions and to do so honestly. However, parents may be called (not as a threat, but as part of understanding the context), and it is usually helpful to clarify calls to them as such.

"When these events happen, our policy is to call parents, and your mom did say that [*target*] had been giving you trouble—can you help me understand more about that?"

Initial Questions Regarding the Threat Incident

1. "Do you know why we are meeting?"
2. "Would you please tell me what happened from your perspective? When did this occur? If I say anything that is not true from your perspective, please let me know. Your perspective on this is what's most important to me right now and I want to understand." [*Adolescents are often sensitive to feeling disrespected, so be sure to convey appropriate respect during your interactions.*]
3. "What exactly was said to/about [*target*]?" [*With greater maturity, adolescents are more likely to provide more context, describing events as "I said ____, but then she said ____, so I then ____," etc.*]
4. "What did you mean/intend when you said/did that?"
5. "How do you think [*target*] reacted/felt/responded to what you said/did?" [*Notice whether the student shows empathy for the target and also remorse. If the student does not show empathy or remorse, that does not mean the punishment or consequences should necessarily be more severe. Rather, consider how the student's circumstances with the target(s) can be altered to impede future events; this sometimes reveals school issues (e.g., bullying that had not been recognized, teachers trying to motivate students by competitions that demoralize the student making threats).*]
6. "Is there anything else going on that led you to feel that way toward [*target*]?" [*Notice forces within or beyond school leading to this threat.*]
7. "How do you feel now about [*target*]? How do you feel about how this played out?" [*Notice if the student is "over" the conflict and whether the student can see different steps to take in future altercations.*]
8. "What is your plan now?} [*Notice whether the student is seeking to make amends and resolve versus justifying statements or actions because of being wronged.*]

If the student resists talking about the incident, the clinician may employ more indirect questions.

1. "Tell me about your classes and teachers this year." [*Notice whether the student has a negative or deteriorating perception of school this year.*]
2. "What parts of school this year have gone well? What do you tend to do during lunch/study periods/unstructured time at school? Is there anyone that you like to hang out with? What do you do for fun?" [*Notice whether the student is enjoying parts of school, is engaged with peers, and is "connected" at school.*]

3. "How do you feel about your schedule this year? What specials/extracurricular activities are you doing?" [*Notice how the student is navigating the school day, getting to and from classes, performing academically, participating in extracurriculars, etc.*]
4. "Are you glad you are at this school? Do you wish anything about this place was different?" [*Notice the student's connection to the school and whether he or she is struggling to find a place versus having given up and being resigned to feeling tormented daily.*]
5. "What is your life like outside school? What do you do at night? Do you spend time with your parents/siblings? How would your parents/siblings describe you if I had just met them? Does anyone else live at home?" [*Notice how the student describes life outside school and connectedness to family.*]

Precipitants to Event

1. "What led up to [*the incident*]?"
2. "Did something happen earlier that led you to [*threat*]?"
3. "Did you feel like you had to [*make the threat*]? Why?"
4. "Has anything else been going on that contributed to this?"
5. "How have you been feeling generally this year?"

Physical Evidence

1. "Did you go online or go out to get anything so that you could actually [hurt/stab/shoot] [*target*]?"
2. "Did you text/e-mail/write/tell anyone about this?"
3. "Do you have a [*weapon*]? Where is it? Have you ever practiced with it? Have you ever used it to protect yourself or in a fight?" [*Notice whether the student expresses aggression toward animals or people.*]

Motives for Behavior

1. "How do you understand what happened?"
2. "What drove/led you to [*incident*]?"
3. "What options did you see or consider? Did you have any options? Why not?"
4. "What did you hope would happen when you said/did [*incident*]?"
5. "Was there anything about [*target*] that made you [*incident*]?"

Plan

1. "How long have the things that bother you been going on that led to [*threat*]?"
2. "What was your plan regarding [*threat*]?"

3. "Did you think about when and where to [*threat*]?"
4. "Did you make plans for how to [*threat*]?"

Accomplices

1. "Did you tell anyone about [*threat*]? Was there anyone you talked to about this?"
2. "Did anyone give you any ideas about what to do?"
3. "Did anyone hear or know about this?"
4. "Did anyone try to stop you from doing this?"
5. "Did anyone suggest other options or solutions to this situation?"

Target(s)

1. "What provoked you to say/do this to [*target*]?"
2. "Did you know you were going to say/do this to [*target*]?" [*Notice whether a particular person mattered.*]
3. "Is there anyone else you feel this way about? Is there anyone else you feel like saying/doing this to?"
4. "Is there something about [*target*] specifically that makes you feel this way?"
5. "Do you still feel this way about [*target*]?"

Weapons

1. "Do you have a [*weapon*]?"
2. "Have you ever used a [*knife, gun, bow, etc.*]? What happened?"
3. "Could you get a [*weapon*] today if you needed one?"
4. "Have you ever used a weapon to hurt anyone?"

Detail Specificity and Plausibility

1. "What did you think would happen when you said/did that?"
2. "What outcome were you most hoping for?"
3. "Had you thought of other things to do/say if this didn't work?"
4. "What other ideas had you considered to get back at/harm [*target*]?"

Emotional Intensity

1. "Were you angry or upset when you said/did [*threat*]?"
2. "Can you remember what you said/did to [*target*]?"
3. "Does anything else get you so upset that you [*incident*]?"
4. "How have you been feeling this year? Has it seemed like other people are trying to make your life hard? Who? Do you know why? How does that make you feel?"

Appendix C

Example Threat Assessment Questions for Use With High School and College Students

Introduction to the Student

Introduce yourself by name and clarify your role (e.g., school counselor, vice principal, provost). Tell the student that you believe that his or her perspective on what happened is important and that you want to understand what happened. Tell the student that you may talk to others (e.g., target, witnesses, parents, teachers) and that he or she will not be forced to tell you anything. Tell the student that he or she can let you know if there is anything he or she is ambivalent about discussing and that you can work together to come up with a solution or decision about what is in the student's best interest.

If the high school or college student shuts down or resists engaging, the clinician can take several steps to increase rapport in an effort to elicit more complete information.

1. "Help me understand the broader context here; how have things proceeded for you here at [*high school/college*]?"
2. "Have things here gone according to plan? If not, what had you anticipated? How do you make sense of how things have gone? Has anything or anyone altered your trajectory?"
3. "What are your interests? Are you planning to study that further down the road or head in a different direction? Are there any causes that are near and dear to you? What do you do for fun?"

Initial Questions Regarding the Threat Incident

1. "Do you know the purpose of our meeting?" [*Notice whether the student is open to discussing the event(s).*]
2. "Please describe to me, in your words, what happened at [*place/time*]." [*Notice the logic leading to the student's actions and whether other unusual events or circumstances may be misperceived or misunderstood.*]
3. "What exactly was said to/about [*target*]?" [*Notice whether comments are more cold and calculated versus hot and "in the moment."*]
4. "What did you mean/intend when you said/did that?"
5. "When did you start feeling this way? Have things happened to make this problem worse?" [*Notice how this situation has been evolving and how much the student is preoccupied with the conflict; this conflict or issue may take up hours of the student's day.*]
6. "How do you think [*target*] reacted/felt/responded to what you said/did? What effect did what you said/did have on [*target*]?" [*Notice any apparent satisfaction the student is deriving from the threat versus persisting fear of the target.*]
7. "Is there anything else going on that led you to feel that way toward [*target*]?" [*Notice the reported sequence of events, the student's perception of others' reactions, and also whether the student is placing everything into one pattern even when it fits poorly.*]
8. "How do you feel now about [*target*]? How do you feel about how this played out?" [*Notice what the student seeks from the target; is it a connection or something closer to annihilation for perceived wrongdoing?*]
9. "What is your plan now?" [*Notice whether the student is seeking resolution or is adhering more rigidly to justifying or defending a position.*]

If the student resists talking about the incident, the clinician may employ more indirect questions.

1. "Tell me about this school; how would you describe this school and what goes on here?" [*Notice how the student perceives the "fairness" and consistency of the school.*]
2. "Is there anyone here you connect with? Do you feel like anyone here really knows you? How would that person describe you?" [*Notice whether the student is "connected" to prosocial others or activities at school.*]
3. "What would you like to be doing after graduation? What do you see yourself doing?"
4. "Is there anything you would change about this school to make it better?"
5. "What do you do when you're not at school? Do you work? Are you engaged in any activities? Do you hang out with anyone outside school? What do you all like to do?"

6. "How are things with your family? How are you getting along with them? Do they get/understand you?" [*Notice changes in family functioning and in parent perceptions of the student.*]
7. "What brings you enjoyment? What kind of people do you like to be around/hang out with?" [*Notice rejection in all life arenas, acceptance by others also nonintegrated at the school, or engagement with others across different groupings and interests.*]

Precipitants to Event

1. "What led up to [*incident*]?"
2. "Did anything else happen that has contributed to [*threat*]?"
3. "What led to this happening now?"
4. "Has this been on your mind for a while?"

Physical Evidence

1. "Did you go online or out to get anything so that you could actually hurt/stab/shoot [*target*]?"
2. "Did you text/e-mail/write/tell anyone about this?"
3. "Do you have a [*weapon*]? Where is it? Have you ever practiced using it? Have you ever used it to defend yourself or in a fight?" [*Notice whether the student expresses aggression toward animals or people.*]

Motives For Behavior

1. "What caused you to [*behavior*]?" [*Notice blaming versus accepting responsibility.*]
2. "What drove/led you to [*incident*]?"
3. "Did you consider other options? What led you to do [*behavior*] instead?"
4. "What did you imagine would happen when you said/did [*incident*]?"
5. "Was there anything about [*target*] that made you [*incident*]?"

Plan

1. "Have you actually planned to do something like what you said/wrote?"
2. "How long have you been thinking about it?"
3. "Have you planned what you would do?"
4. "Where did you get your ideas to [*incident*]?"
5. "How long have you been thinking about that?"
6. "Had you had other ideas or plans?"

7. "Had you tried to do anything before? Did something not work with that plan?"

Accomplices

1. "Did you tell anyone about [*threat*]? Was there anyone you talked to about this?"
2. "Did you ask anyone or get any ideas elsewhere about what to do?"
3. "Did anyone hear or know about this?"
4. "Did anyone try to stop you from doing this?"
5. "Did anyone suggest something else to do?"

Target(s)

1. "Did you know you were going to say/do this to [*target*]?" [*Notice whether a particular person mattered.*]
2. "What led you to say/do this to [*target*]?"
3. "Is there anyone else you feel this way about? Is there anyone else you feel like saying/doing this to?"
4. "Is there something about [*target*] specifically that makes you feel this way?"
5. "How do you feel now about [*target*]?"

Weapons

1. "Do you have [*weapons*]?"
2. "Have you ever used a [*knife, gun, bow, etc.*]? What happened?"
3. "Could you get a [*weapon*] today if you needed one?"
4. "Have you ever used a weapon to hurt anyone?"

Detail Specificity/Plausibility

1. "What did you think would happen when you said/did [*behavior*]?"
2. "What were you most hoping for when you said/did [*behavior*]?"
3. "Had you thought of other things to do/say if this didn't work?"
4. "What other ideas had you considered to get back at/harm [*target*]?"

Emotional Intensity

1. "Were you angry or upset when you said/did [*threat*]?"
2. "What do you remember saying/doing to [*target*]?"
3. "Does anything or anyone else get you upset as much as [*target*]?"
4. "How has your emotional health been this year? Has it been different this year? How is it better or worse than last year?"

Index

Page numbers printed in **boldface** type refer to tables, figures, or boxes.